TERRY RUMMIN

So, I've got Parkinson's Disease

Matador
9 Priory Business Park
Kibworth Beauchamp
Leicestershire LE8 0RX, UK
Tel: (+44) 116 279 2299
Fax: (+44) 116 279 2277
Email: books@troubador.co.uk
Web: www.troubador.co.uk/matador

ISBN 978 1780883 755

British Library Cataloguing in Publication Data.
A catalogue record for this book is available from the British Library.

Printed and bound in the UK by TJ International, Padstow, Cornwall

Matador is an imprint of Troubador Publishing Ltd

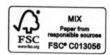

For Jack, who has been with me all the way.

To Mary and John for caring, over many years.

And to all the many people who have put up with my enthusiasm and doggedness about this book.

CONTENTS

CONTENTS

1
THE START

When I was first diagnosed with Parkinson's I didn't know what to feel. That sounds a bit odd, especially coming from a psychologist, but feelings are tied up with expectations and I didn't know what to expect from Parkinson's. I veered wildly between visualising myself in a wheelchair within a few months and not really believing that there was anything wrong with me. I am hoping that writing this book and describing my experience so far will be useful to other people who have been diagnosed with Parkinson's, to help them with their expectations of how the condition may affect them. Having said that; although people with Parkinson's have a lot in common, their experiences can also be very different and it is quite likely that some of what I have experienced and what has helped me will not be relevant to others. However, that is the nub of the challenge of having Parkinson's. You have to build up a new, individual understanding of yourself. Unlike the case with many other medical ailments, you have to become an expert about yourself!

Anyway, to start my story, I was officially diagnosed with Parkinson's Disease eight years ago, but I now recognise that I already had it at least two years prior to this. Also my husband says that with the help of hindsight, he can recall symptoms a few years before that. As I write this, it seems that I have had Parkinson's for about ten years. I have worked full-time for all this period and only recently decided that I was ready for retirement. I will not pretend that it has always been easy to continue working, especially recently, but it has certainly been possible and very important for me, my family and hopefully for the people with and for whom I have worked. I have been a counselling psychologist and an educational psychologist. Over the past eight years I have run a team of educational psychologists, have assessed a large number of children and young people with regard to their special educational needs, have lectured and given talks and have worked as a counsellor and as a supervisor for trainee counsellors and experienced counsellors. In the last two years my work has taken me to various parts of the country.

I would wish to encourage others to keep working, if they want to work. Working is one of the ways we gain and maintain our self-respect in this society and, thanks to recent Disability Discrimination legislation, we all have the right to work, even if we have a disability and even if some adjustments have to be made to enable us to work. Finding out that one has Parkinson's could precipitate a person into seeking early retirement out of a lack of understanding. Equally, the ignorance of what Parkinson's is about, could encourage employers to get rid of employees who may then lose out, not only on material benefits such as pension rights but also psychologically, in the areas of self confidence and self-esteem. A friend told me a long time ago that he never made major decisions when angry or depressed. In the case of Parkinson's and whether to carry on working, that seems very good advice to follow.

My first awareness of having a problem, which eventually turned out to be Parkinson's, was an increasing shaking in my right arm. I had been stressed, owing to the serious illness of one of my sons and assumed that the stress had caused the shaking. I tried all the ways of helping myself that I could think of: I went to my GP; I referred myself to Occupational Health at work; I visited an acupuncturist for several sessions; I visited a homeopath, a naturopath and a hypnotherapist. Each time I referred myself to a new person, we would both gaze at my arm, which was showing an increasing liveliness, then the prescribed intervention was made and after various lapses of time we would gaze at my arm again. Disappointingly to me, but it seemed not to my arm which continued shaking with energetic enthusiasm, none of the interventions worked, although I certainly enjoyed the hypnotherapy which induced a wonderful feeling of calm and I was given a lot of helpful nutritional advice from the naturopath. In contrast, I remember the last of my five sessions at the acupuncture clinic: my arm was placed on a white cushion and contemplated by two acupuncturists and me. Then the recommended treatment was carried out, which consisted of acupuncture in one of my ears and which was extremely painful. At the end of the session all three of us contemplated my arm again as it lay on its white cushion. But in rebellious defiance the arm shook more than ever. I was told by the defeated acupuncturists that I must have had a small stroke and that this would be causing the shaking.… I was not convinced. I was also unimpressed by the homeopath: the person concerned dangled a sort of crystal over my wrist, came to some conclusions and gave me one tablet to take. This should really help the shaking, I was told. But there was one proviso; I must only take this tablet in safe conditions because it might cause a dramatic reaction. So I carefully took the tablet, waited and…experienced nothing at all.

These people to whom I had turned for help had been personally recommended to me and no doubt were useful for others, but my problem remained and I was becoming more in need of a solution. I even gave up coffee, joined a gym and, more importantly exercised at the gym three times per week. But still my arm kept shaking.

I visited my GP every so often and he was interested and sympathetic. After a while he made a diagnosis of 'familial tremor' and he recommended beta-blockers. A familial tremor is a tremor of unknown origin, which runs in families. The beta-blockers helped a little but by now I was developing another symptom; my writing was becoming smaller and untidier. I had always been proud of my large, I felt decisive, readable script but not any more. Secretaries, who had congratulated me in the past on the clarity of my writing, now peered and frowned at my written offerings, turning them around in the air in front of their eyes, to try to make sense of them. Little did I know that 'micrographia' is a sign of Parkinson's. And there were other symptoms such as becoming very cold, to the point of shivering, which of course enhanced the shaking arm. I noticed that I became particularly cold in stressful situations and prepared for them by wearing extra clothes and turning up the heating. One symptom, of which I was not aware but which a psychiatrist colleague later told me he had noticed, was a tendency to clench my right hand in a kind of fist, with the thumb held between my forefinger and second finger. The technical term for this is a 'pill-rolling tremor' because the person may look as though they are rolling a pill between their thumb and first two fingers. Strangely enough, I remember another colleague commenting to me over twenty-five years earlier on my habit of apparently unconsciously clenching my right hand in a fist.

Eighteen months went by and all the above symptoms increased in severity, but I did not view them as being linked and part of some larger picture. For example, I did not perceive the shaking and the small writing as being related. I perceived them as being separate from each other as of course I would have done, not knowing anything much about Parkinson's. As before, if I had had to put these unusual behaviours down to anything, it would have been to stress: by now my first son's condition had improved greatly but my second son was then taken seriously ill, from a different although equally serious condition from the first son.

My doctor referred me to a consultant. So, on a cold day in February I sat with the consultant and Jack, my husband, in one of the big London hospitals. The consultant had taken my case history, had asked me to walk up and down the room, to open and close my thumb and fore-fingers rapidly and to write 'Mary had a little Lamb' over and over again. At the end of all this he said, 'Well Terry, I expect you know what I am going to diagnose?' I nodded in agreement, thinking, 'Yes, stress.' But, what he said was, 'You have Parkinson's Disease; a degenerative neurological condition, which will never improve, will get steadily worse and for which there is no cure'. Both our mouths fell open as Jack and I gazed at the consultant, who must have been unnerved by our responses. 'Oh,' he continued, 'you weren't prepared for this diagnosis'. The consultant recommended some medication and suggested he refer me to another consultant in order, it seemed, that I would have the opportunity of seeing the same person at each of my appointments. However, I did not take in much of this part of the interview!

I did understand, however, from what the consultant said, that I had no swing in my right arm when I walked and that my ability to carry out repeated fine motor movements with my right hand was diminishing. These, together with the tremor and the increasingly small writing, were symptoms of Parkinson's Disease.

I was silent as we returned home on the Underground. So was Jack. He told me later that he was thinking that we would cope with Parkinson's, whatever the implications. As for me, I was really surprised to have been diagnosed with the condition.

2
OTHER PEOPLE

I must have been in a state of shock at first but, on the surface, I carried on as normal. I hugged my new knowledge to myself for a few days, vaguely aware that telling people my news would change their perception of me.

The first person I told was my boss. She was extremely kind. I then visited Occupational Health and told them. The person I talked to apologised for their Service not having considered Parkinson's when I had referred myself to them. I found myself reassuring her. I then told my team of psychologists and the secretarial team. I told other people with whom I came into contact through work. When I had to address a large group of people, as in a training session, I would mention at the beginning of the session that the reason I shook was because I had Parkinson's. I told my friends and of course I told my family. Although at first I occasionally found it harrowing to tell people that I had Parkinson's, I rapidly felt better for bringing the situation out into the open. I have asked myself why I was so 'up-front' about it all from the start. The main answer is, I think, that I have always felt a compulsion to face up to the worst things that have happened to me, as soon as possible, so that I can then try to do something about them. Also, I was meeting with many members of the public as part of my work and I wanted to accustom myself as soon as possible to talking about the Parkinson's in as natural a way as I could, so as not to become overwhelmed in public. Then there was the fact that, as a psychologist, one is always meeting with people who have problems; it seemed incongruous to me, to expect other people to face up to their own problems whilst avoiding mine. Finally, I have always been very interested in the whole area of counselling and I believe that openness and honesty are integral to counselling. So, if I had kept the Parkinson's to myself, I would have been concealing something that was becoming a core part of me. I always let people know that I had Parkinson's, if they rang me to ask for professional help and had not met with me before.

I have found it very helpful to bring the subject of Parkinson's to the fore and to try to cope with it in that way. Although I understand that some people would prefer not to discuss their disability, in my case I prefer to talk about it.

In my work as an educational psychologist, I have told my clients about my having Parkinson's on first meeting with them, whether they are children, young people or adults, including parents, carers and school staff. I soon found that my shaking became more noticeable and other symptoms became obvious and I didn't want the client to feel uncertain or concerned about these. I have found that with adults my information has often acted as an icebreaker; people frequently telling me about relatives or friends with Parkinson's. Children have often reacted with interest and questions and, needless to say, those with behavioural problems are generally the most interested and the most helpful. For once they are not the one with the imperfections!

In fact, I have generally become more aware of the importance of imperfection. Psychologists don't usually claim to be perfect, but they often have this expectation thrust upon them and they can then be blamed for not living up to it. However, I am so obviously imperfect that often a relaxed atmosphere can be established, in which the other person has the opportunity to give to me, as well as my giving to them. I do not think I exaggerate when I state that we move away from the 'expert / lay person' situation, into a more equal sharing of power.

An area which I feel has benefited from my obvious imperfections has been my assessments of very disabled children and young people. On some occasions I feel that I have acted as a role model in those situations.

But not everyone is positive of course and when I have experienced negative reactions to my informing people that I have Parkinson's Disease, I have found that I have had to adjust, not only to having Parkinson's, but also to the responses of these people to my having Parkinson's and to their effect on my self-esteem.

In the early days I had many kind phone calls and messages, but one particular phone call illustrates the interesting ambivalence which misfortune in others evokes in some people. An acquaintance rang me to express sympathy about my condition. The person seemed very concerned and so I reassured them that there were drugs I could take, that a lot of research was happening, that things were not so bad. Still my acquaintance bemoaned my situation. Eventually I said, 'Well, at least it's not life threatening'.

'Oh, I think it is,' was the answer.

I tell this story with amusement but, as with all humour, it illustrates the shadow side of human nature as well as evoking an explosion of laughter at the ridiculous. One may well ask how anybody could be tactless enough to suggest to someone with a recently diagnosed serious condition, who is obviously trying to be positive, that things may be even worse than she thinks.

What I had to try to understand was that some people (a small minority) did not want me to be positive, did not want me to overcome my problem, and did not want me to succeed in the face of adversity. And just as some people didn't want me to succeed, some parts of myself also wanted to give up on me. From a theoretical point of view, I was not surprised. I knew that it is part of being human to have a negative side as well as a positive side. The important thing for me was to recognise the negativity in myself and to try not to attribute it completely to others. There was very little I could do about other people's destructive feelings towards me, but there was a lot I could do about my own destructive feelings towards myself. Of course this applies to us all, Parkinson's or no Parkinson's.

As I gradually develop into what is called a disabled person I have found that it has not been the blatant prejudice shown by a very few people against disability that has tested my self-confidence. Lawyers are there to deal with that. The enemy within is far more insidious; the creeping self-doubt, which claims to be caused by other people's occasional thoughtless remarks, but is more likely to be because of my own lack of confidence about myself as a human being, now that my outer image is so obviously flawed.

I have been full of admiration for those people who genuinely still perceive me as being myself, whatever my outward presentation is like. As for those people who have really seemed to value my skills, my personality or whatever, and actually need them, well they are worth more than I can express. They make me feel that I really am still me.

A person who has a developing disability is in danger of losing their self-confidence and even their sense of self and I have been just as susceptible to doing so, as anyone else. No amount of psychological knowledge protects me from feeling inadequate when I can't do some of the simple things that others can do and, even more importantly, that I used to be able to do. One of the ways in which we define ourselves is in terms of how we think others perceive us. The naturally shy person cringes at the thought of crossing a crowded room because they think that they know what the umpteen pairs of eyes are perceiving and the umpteen brains are thinking. In fact, this hypothetical shy person is mistaken in assuming that they can know such things for sure about other people, let alone that these perceptions are negative. The way out of their shyness is for the person to become genuinely self-conscious, not in the usual sense of the term, but in the sense of becoming conscious of the person they are. Then the state of mind of the person crossing the room is not a reflection of what they think others are thinking, but of whom they know they are.

Someone helped me a lot by telling me about how she had once developed a serious allergic reaction, which had caused her face to swell up in a very unsightly manner. Every time she had met someone new she had wanted to say to them, 'I am not really like this. This is only temporary.'

This person said to me that she imagined that was what I wanted to say to people and I agreed.

But the truth is that I am now really like this and crossing the chasm between hankering after the old me and accepting the new me is the equivalent achievement of the once shy person now crossing the room with their head held high and even cracking a joke on the way.

No, I don't think I have attained such self-acceptance yet, but I won't stop trying!

3
THEORY

One of the things I did immediately I knew I had Parkinson's Disease was to learn about it. I joined the Parkinson's Society and read the information it published. I read books written by people with Parkinson's. I visited the medical sections of eminent bookshops and bought the most up to date books I could find on Parkinson's. In these ways I have built up a fund of knowledge about the condition and I have found this invaluable in interpreting my symptoms as they have developed, in understanding the effects of the drugs I have taken for Parkinson's and in trying to distinguish between whether a symptom is drug-induced or Parkinson's induced. Initially, I had no idea of the importance of this distinction but I have found that at times my drugs have caused me problems, which I had originally put down to Parkinson's; for example, suffering from 'frequency', a term used to describe the need to keep passing urine. I have also used the knowledge I have acquired, to decide on which prescribed drugs to agree to take and which to defer, at least for the time being.

I have learned that in the UK, about 2 in 100 people are likely to develop Parkinson's Disease during their lifetime*. It usually starts at around fifty to sixty years old, but it can start earlier and some young people in their teens have been diagnosed with Parkinson's. It is a little more prevalent in men than in women and you are extremely unlikely to develop Parkinson's if you smoke! Some people have suggested, although it has not been proven, that there is such a thing as the Parkinson's personality; a rather rigid, non-addictive personality. (Well, I have to admit that I must have been one of a minority who lived through the sixties and never took a 'recreational drug'. Also, I have smoked approximately four cigarettes in my life and certainly didn't inhale them. But 'rigid' ? I don't like to admit to the negative implications of this attribute, but I do stick relentlessly to such things as professional ethics. Yes, some people might describe me as rigid…but they would be exaggerating, of course!)

No one has as yet ascertained the cause of Parkinson's. There are some rare forms, which run in families, but generally speaking it seems that Parkinson's occurs as a result of the interaction between environmental factors and some unknown genetic propensities. As regards the environmental factors, pesticides are currently one of the popular suspects. (I lived in Malta for part of my childhood and on many occasions there I walked through clouds of what I was told was DDT, a very strong pesticide, whose use has now been banned.)

Whatever the reason for developing Parkinson's, the effect is that vital cells in the brain, which produce a substance called dopamine, are destroyed. By the time the person notices that they have symptoms of Parkinson's, their dopamine levels have fallen to 20% of normal*. So far, no one has found a way of preventing this. Dopamine is one of various substances called neurotransmitters.

Neurotransmitters facilitate the passing of messages along nerve cells in the brain to the rest of the body. So, because I lack the amount of dopamine I need, various messages don't get from my brain through to various parts of my body and hence my symptoms.

That is an ultra-simplified account of Parkinson's disease and it is obviously quite inadequate, but I am not trying to write a medical book. There are many interesting sources of information about the brain, nerve cells and neuro-transmitters which one can access in libraries, good bookshops and on the Internet.

It is difficult for the medical people to diagnose Parkinson's disease in the early stages because it can be confused with other conditions, but it is generally agreed that if one has one or two of the following symptoms then Parkinson's is a possible diagnosis:

- Tremor (although a quarter of Parkinson's sufferers don't shake);

- Bradykinesis (slowness and diminished movement);

- Stiffness and possible rigidity;

- Postural disturbance (physical unsteadiness and instability).

Parkinson's Disease is named after James Parkinson, the son of an apothecary, who was born in the eighteenth century and who described the condition, in an essay published in 1817, having observed it in several people. For a long time there was no medical remedy for

Parkinson's and so the patient's symptoms simply intensified as the disease progressed.

However, since the 1970s, fairly effective medications have been developed which aim to minimise the symptoms of Parkinson's. Because the disease results from a lack of dopamine, the main method of treating Parkinson's has been to attempt to replace the lost dopamine. Unfortunately, the body cannot cope with neat dopamine but it can turn another chemical into dopamine. This chemical is the one that comes before dopamine (its precursor) in a particular chemical pathway and is called levodopa. Thus levodopa develops into dopamine, given the right physiological environment.

There are drawbacks to the intake of levodopa, however. One is that a few years down the line, if one has been taking it regularly, one is likely to develop involuntary movements called dyskinesias. Yes, and these are in addition to the Parkinson's symptoms! Another problem about levodopa is that it is enthusiastically broken down by the digestive system so that only a little of what levodopa one ingests is made available for the brain. There has been progress in recent years in the development of drugs which slow the breakdown of levodopa, but still the greater percentage of it is destroyed by the body. That little remaining bit of levodopa is of vital importance to Parkinson's sufferers, however. After it has heroically negotiated what scientists call the 'blood-brain barrier' (a 21st century physiological equivalent of the Berlin wall?) the small amount of resultant dopamine can do its job and for a time the various Parkinson's symptoms recede, more or less, depending on the individual's particular response to levodopa.

It all sounds 'hit and miss' and this is because everything depends on how one's body physiology works. The doctor or consultant can only do their best to give the patient a general description of the efficiency and side effects of Parkinson's drugs. They cannot accurately predict individual people's reactions. That is why it is so important to take notice of how one reacts to various drugs. For example, I currently take levodopa and I have found that I do not react well to eating protein close in time to taking the levodopa. I shall describe this in more detail in Chapter Seven.

Although levodopa is a very successful drug and I dread to think how Parkinson's sufferers coped in the past without it, it has its down sides, as mentioned above and a few people cannot tolerate it at all. Hence, in recent times there has been an all-out effort to develop drugs which mimic the effects of levodopa, but which don't have its major side effects. These drugs are called dopamine agonists and if one starts taking these early on in the development of Parkinson's, then the introduction of levodopa can often be delayed, hence delaying the possibility of its major side effects such as the involuntary movements mentioned above, which can be intrusive and socially embarrassing.

One recent thrust of research is directed towards encouraging the Parkinson's sufferer to develop his or her own dopamine producing cells. This research relies on the availability of sufficient stem cells. Another direction of research aims to slow down the degeneration of the nerve cells that produce dopamine.

All the technical books stress that the development of Parkinson's differs from person to person and so it is not possible in most cases to give a clear prognosis. However, the factors in one's favour are good general health and a positive attitude.

Unfortunately, up to 50% of people with Parkinson's become clinically depressed*. Depression is of course an understandable reaction to being diagnosed with an incurable condition, but it is also thought that in some cases the depression can be a result of the chemical changes in the brain, associated with Parkinson's. Luckily, depression can be ameliorated, whether by therapy or drugs or both.

References:
* Tugwell C. *Parkinson's Disease in Focus*, 2008,
Pharmaceutical Press, London

4
AN IMPORTANT FACT

I have learned the theory about Parkinson's from books and journals, but I have also had the benefit of a practical course as the condition has progressed in myself. From this I have learned some major facts about Parkinson's.

The main, most important lesson has been to abandon physical effort and physical perseverance as a technique for getting things done. I have had to let go of my favourite method for tackling life's challenges, which used to be a selection of variations on the theme of, 'if at first you don't succeed, try, try, try again'. This had served me well since being a child. For example, I moved school frequently as a child because my family moved from place to place and sometimes from country to country. I had to cope with a frequently changing school curriculum and in one case a change of language as well as the whole social upheaval which moving home entailed. I also had child-minding and housekeeping responsibilities, being the oldest of several brothers and sisters. The way I managed was to keep trying, not to give up, to keep chipping away at challenges, to persevere, to work harder etc… Many of the efforts I made were physical in that they involved time, physical effort and physical perseverance. I was sure that almost anything was possible if I worked hard enough. Today I find such a whole-hearted commitment to this strategy questionable from a psychological point of view but it was my strategy for years and it served me well.

However, with Parkinson's, trying and then trying again, let alone trying for a third time is likely to leave me exhausted, dispirited and vanquished. Parkinson's has no respect for the Protestant work ethic. An illustration of this is in my motor skills: writing, cutting with scissors, peeling vegetables, drying after a bath or shower, dressing and undressing, cleaning my teeth, straightening a pile of papers, getting money out of a purse, putting objects into a bag, cutting food, are all examples of tasks I find difficult. I can list many other such motor difficulties: I cannot aim or direct objects accurately; I drop things; I cannot hold things firmly with my right hand; if I repeat movements they slow down. In short, I am extremely clumsy. I also tire readily. But I become even clumsier and totally exhausted if I persist in trying to achieve a physical task that I am finding difficult. It is far better for me to give in straight away and to look for another way around the problem. I give examples below of some of the alternatives I have used:

WRITING.
Alternative:
Use a laptop computer.

CUTTING OUT.
Alternative:
Ask someone if they will do it for me.

PEELING VEGETABLES.
Alternative:
Use a 'magic peeler'. This is a peeler with a rocking blade

20

that has a double cutting edge. The device has transformed my life.

DRYING AFTER A BATH OR SHOWER.
Alternative:
Use a towelling bath-robe.

CLEANING TEETH.
Alternative:
Use an electric toothbrush.

DRESSING
Alternative:
Take the time necessary; get all the clothes ready in one place; ensure that none are inside out; use a full-length mirror to help with zips and buttons. After putting on each garment, sit down and take a short break.

UNDRESSING
Alternative:
This is hard, particularly at night because of extra tiredness. I have found that my best strategy is to enthuse myself about getting undressed by visualising how nice it will be to sit in bed, propped up by a pillow and reading a good book. Otherwise I tend to get slower and slower...

STRAIGHTENING A PILE OF PAPERS.
Alternative:
It has to be one piece of paper at a time, carefully. There is no short cut.

GETTING MONEY OUT OF A PURSE.
Alternative:
Use a purse that is easy to open and close; fold up notes

singly in preparation; only have a few coins in the purse and know which they are. Try to keep calm at checkouts. If necessary, I explain to the person behind me that I have Parkinson's and hope they understand that's why I am holding up the queue.

PUTTING OBJECTS INTO A BAG OR BRIEFCASE.
Alternative:
Again, keep calm; prop up the bag; slowly and deliberately put one object into the bag at a time; on no account do I allow myself to be rushed.

EATING.
Alternative:
Buy an extremely sharp knife and use it instead of an ordinary dinner knife; use a spoon; use fingers; eat risotto when out for a meal. (In fact I think it should become obligatory for all restaurants to provide a risotto option because it is so easy to eat for people like me). If necessary my husband cuts up all the food on his plate and then we do a discrete swap.

The point I am trying to emphasise is that having Parkinson's has taught me that putting more and more physical effort into an activity is the equivalent of banging my head against a brick wall. It is pointless. Instead I have needed to develop a creative approach, whereby I have accepted that the usual way I have tackled a task no longer works or is too tiring and I have come up with an alternative way of achieving the task.

My most spectacular success has been in finding a new

way of getting off the floor or out of the bath. The usual way of getting up out of these positions does not work for me and leads to my resembling a stranded, upside down tortoise. The more I make an effort, the more I get nowhere. However, if I turn onto my hands and knees I can get off the floor or out of the bath with what I feel is quite an agile movement. If I am on my own and find it difficult to get out of a low chair I will move onto the floor, onto my hands and knees and then get up in the manner described above. However, I am a little embarrassed at doing this in public. Somehow I can't raise the confidence to slip gracefully to my knees in a crowded underground train, prior to getting out at the next stop. Still, that might be better than being left behind, as I recently discovered, when Jack, my husband, turned to me on leaving the train and found that I wasn't there… I was still trying to drag myself out of the seat!

One of the alternative strategies I have mentioned above is to ask someone to help. When one develops a disability one can be reluctant to ask for help but that overlooks the fact that helping can often be as useful to the helper as to the helped. So this is a strategy not to be ignored. Friends are very ready to lend a hand and strangers have probably already deduced that there is a problem. After all, most of us would help if asked, so why wouldn't someone else?

All the methods given above are designed to minimise or change the nature of my physical effort. As I've already indicated, Parkinson's has no respect for effort or repetition. If I repeat activities I become worse at them and then exhausted. The exhaustion has to be felt, in order to be really appreciated. It's not just the tiredness I have felt in the past after a strenuous day; it has a quality of final desperation about it. As I have summoned my last quantum of energy to pull up my trousers in the ladies' loo and as I have been conscious of the waiting queue outside, at times I have wanted to give up … but I have not yet found a toilet worth giving up in and anyway there is the rest of my life waiting outside the door.

Parkinson's is the antithesis of forced, hurried movement and, as I have already said, Parkinson's certainly does not approve of repetitive movements. One of the tests I am given every time I see my consultant is to repeat a particular hand movement and the more I repeat the movement, the more I slow down.

Sometimes, if I become very tired, I just feel like keeping still, even standing still and letting the world go by. Parkinson's approves of this.

5
STRESS

Another fact that I have clearly understood since my Parkinson's has developed is that there really is nothing worth getting stressed about. That is a cliché and a truism of course, but in this case it is meant far more literally than is usual. Stress involves the production of noradrenaline and adrenaline, which are hormones and neuro-transmitters. Dopamine is the precursor to noradrenaline and noradrenaline is the precursor to adrenaline. (As mentioned previously, a precursor in a physiological pathway is the chemical produced immediately prior to another chemical.) So, the production of adrenaline, because it uses up dopamine, further depletes the Parkinson's sufferer's meagre store of dopamine. Less dopamine means even less capability of doing the things I want to do, like putting on my jacket or signing my name. So, getting stressed is literally, physically, not worth it.

Some time ago, when I had finished some College training work, one of the people in charge said to me that she had admired my calm attitude throughout. I was pleased and thanked her for her remark. When I thought about it, I realised that my calmness was a direct result of my trying to manage Parkinson's. In institutional life one can get used to reacting with a sense of urgency to what are often not genuinely urgent situations. There is almost an obligation to panic. Well, I can't afford to panic. If I do, then some of my small stock of dopamine will convert itself to noradrenaline and then to adrenaline and I will have even more difficulty in pulling up my trousers in the ladies' loo. So, I have tried to develop an attitude towards panic-encouraging situations, which says, 'I won't'. I try to be resolutely firm about this, first with myself and then, if necessary, with others.

For the same reason, I have tried to give up getting involved in heated discussions or becoming pointlessly irritated with people or worrying about things which I cannot alter. I can thank Parkinson's for these changes in myself, to the extent that I have achieved them. I am not saying that it is easy to alter one's habits, but it is possible, especially if the stakes are high enough.

I was recently reminded that I am not always as calm as I would like to be, when I requested holiday insurance to cover me for a visit to France.

My request was made by phone. Because I have Parkinson's I was put through to someone with a medical checklist who asked me various questions. I could visualise my dopamine turning into noradrenaline, and then into adrenaline, as I tried to answer three of the questions in particular.

The employee at the other end asked me whether my condition had deteriorated in the last year. I explained that Parkinson's is a deteriorating condition. The person at the other end asked if that was a 'yes' or a 'no'. I explained again and the questioner went to talk to his supervisor. He returned and said that the supervisor said the answer had to be a 'yes' or a 'no'.

The next question asked whether I had any undiagnosed medical conditions. After checking that I had not misheard, I pointed out that I would not know if I had any undiagnosed conditions, but I thought it likely that many of us would be in that situation. The person at the other end asked if that was a 'yes' or a 'no'.

The final question was then asked: Would I be willing to pay a purely voluntary contribution of just over nine pounds, the implication being that this was for administration work. The person at the other end stressed that the contribution was voluntary. I asked what would happen if I did not pay this. The answer given was that I would not receive the insurance.

By then I was definitely losing dopamine to adrenaline. I decided that this was a game that I had to play, gave the 'right' answers, including the one about the 'voluntary' contribution, and quitted the conversation as soon as I could. I thought about ringing the managers and complaining, but at that time, feeling as I did, I would only have become more stressed had I done so.

I have found several ways to become more relaxed and have listed them below.

1. Practise relaxation techniques.

Mine involves lying on my back in a symmetrical position on the floor or other flat surface, concentrating on breathing in and out and mentally saying to myself, 'arms relaxed', 'legs relaxed' etc… throughout all the parts of my body. I mentally say the part of my body on the in breath and 'relaxed' on the out breath. I find that if I do this for about five minutes per day, I feel a real difference. There are various books and tapes on sale which teach relaxation, as do many counsellors and therapists. Some people prefer to practise meditation and I understand that it can give the same kind of result.

2. Get more rest.

As I have already indicated, Parkinson's makes you tired. Tiredness impedes physical functioning and that causes stress. In my case I feel better if I don't get up too early in the morning or if I have an afternoon nap. Presumably, I may one day need both. Incidentally, since taking levodopa my sleep has greatly improved and I remember my dreams far more than I did in the past.

3. Get to know what constitutes a really relaxing environment for oneself and increase one's exposure to it.

For example, recently I have been lucky enough to spend some months in France in a country area and have really enjoyed the relaxation brought about by the lack of traffic and the country pace of life. Not that one has to go to another country to find an environment that is personally relaxing. I have a friend who loves being outdoors and walks up to fifteen miles a day to preserve her equanimity. No, she doesn't have Parkinson's but the point is that she has found what is right for her. Some people like looking at the sea. Others meditate. Others find peace in their stamp albums. The nature of the activity doesn't matter. Whether it is personally relaxing is what matters and now is the time to indulge oneself.

4. Learn to recognise personal causes of stress.

That sounds simple, but it does involve thinking time and a good friend or counsellor. They will be able to point out situations that cause one stress even when one is denying the fact. The reason for this denial is frequently because one feels that one 'shouldn't' find such situations stressful. It is important to remember that no one can help what they feel. What is important is to be truthful with ourselves concerning our feelings and to aim to look after ourselves.

5. Avoid situations that cause stress.

Again, this is easier to say than to do but when the options come down to shaking more and moving less, versus bringing some change into my life, I would definitely choose the latter. There are, of course, some stressful situations that one can't avoid, but these are probably less in number than one assumes before looking closely at them.

6. Learn to say no without feeling guilty.

What I found most difficult at first about avoiding stressful situations was saying 'no' and feeling selfish for doing so. In the past I would usually manage to fit extra things into what was always a busy schedule, particularly if these things involved people. I suppose that my first step forward was to say 'no', *despite* feeling guilty, bearing in mind that the physical repercussions to myself would not be worth saying 'yes'. After doing this on many occasions, it has become easier. However, I still feel a bit of a kill-joy when I go home early because I am tired or choose to read a book rather than go out.

7. Being with people whose company is good for me.

As regards social situations there are people with whom it is good for me to spend time. I come away from them feeling more whole and happier. These are the people with whom I opt to be. There are various reasons for why one opts to be with people who have the opposite effect and these usually boil down to a sense of duty. However, it is likely that if one spends time with someone, simply because of a sense of duty, this will result in a sterile experience for the other person as much as for oneself. If someone makes me feel drained, then they are not good for me and I am sure that I am not good for them. I must stress that this applies to social situations and not to counselling or supervision work, where other criteria apply.

8. Letting go of resentments, whether these are criticisms of oneself or of other people or of 'fate'.

Constantly feeling negative does not make for relaxation. I try to remember that, like others, I am a mixture of good and bad, positive and negative and that it is a waste of my time to ruminate over situations where I could have acted better or when other people have treated me unfairly. Some people perceive contracting a disease such as Parkinson's as a sort of punishment for how they have lived their lives.

The light-hearted response to such an assertion is that, if that is so, then it is surprising that the whole population hasn't got Parkinson's. A more serious response would be, however, that such self-blame could be a sign of depression and should be taken seriously.

9. Having a plan.

I find that making a plan, either to deal with a difficult situation or to achieve a wished for outcome, gives me hope and confidence, helps me to feel in control of myself and certainly relaxes me. With Parkinson's, it is important to retain as much flexibility and choice over one's life as possible because one is inevitably faced with losing control over certain areas.

10. Having fun.

Enjoying oneself, laughing, looking at the funny sides of life are all important in putting things in perspective and keeping one relaxed. I think that funny people deserve sainthoods and I welcome them into my life, whether in person or in books, films, television programmes or by any other means.

6
A PARADOX

There is one very surprising fact I have learned from having Parkinson's. At least it was surprising to me when I first realised it because it seemed to fly in the face of logic and because it required that I develop a fresh perspective.

The issue in question is around simple and complex activities:

There are some activities, which I have routinely perceived as being fairly basic and simple for myself, such as washing or eating. In contrast, there are activities that I would perceive as requiring far more complex skills from myself, such as giving a talk or writing a detailed report. Further, I know that I mastered the basic skills before developing the more complex ones. So if the basic skills were lost I started to assume that the more complex ones would definitely be threatened.

To explain further, let me put all this in context. I had been feeling embarrassed when eating out because of not being able to cut up some foods, shaking whilst using the knife, fork or spoon, finding it difficult to get up from the table and swerving as I walked out of the café or restaurant, hence probably confirming people's suspicions that I was tipsy! Because I regarded going out for a meal as a fairly fundamental activity for myself and because I seemed to be failing at it, this coloured my view of myself in general and I expected the same kind of failure in all the tasks I carried out and certainly in the more complex tasks. This made me feel quite despondent.

But I was comparing unlike categories, which cannot be compared. My table manners are one thing, whereas my ability to give talks is another. Similarly, my face flannel technique is one thing and my ability to write reports is another. Assuming that I was generally becoming worse at everything because I was getting worse at some things was understandable from an emotional point of view, but was logically misguided. It was understandable emotionally because any loss, including losing some of our physical abilities, is like a bereavement and being bereaved churns up all sorts of negative feelings including lowering of self-esteem. But looking at the situation logically rather than emotionally, I didn't have to lose confidence. For example, there was no reason, unless I wanted to give demonstrations of table etiquette, why my deteriorating restaurant technique should affect my ability to give talks.

In fact, in the area of giving talks I found that having Parkinson's actually improved my performance. Because my shaking did not facilitate the use of PowerPoint or holding a sheaf of notes in my hand, I became used to giving my talks without notes. I developed methods for remembering without the prompt of notes. For example, I became used to dividing my talk into chunks and numbering them. Then I would visualise a string with numbers along it and when giving the talk I would mentally proceed along the piece of string to deliver all the parts of the talk. Consequently, I became far more sensitive to the audience's reaction and could pick up on people's expressions and comments more flexibly. This was because I now had a greater attention span available to notice people's responses whilst it was not being taken up with trying to keep track of notes or adhering rigidly to a previously prepared PowerPoint schedule.

So, I came to understand the fact that, just because I can't do simple things doesn't mean that I can't do complex things.

However, one might say that comparing my table manners with my ability to give a talk is unfair because they are obviously such different abilities. I might have agreed had I not also discovered areas where it seems that I am using the same basic skills, but in some cases I can manage or am improving, whereas in others I am definitely deteriorating. Take for example my handwriting and my typing.

I have already described how my writing became smaller and smaller. This continued and apart from a short period about an hour and a quarter after taking levodopa (I will explain this later) my writing has become almost illegible after a few words.

So, I largely stopped using writing to communicate and took to the laptop. This involves typing with both hands and I would have expected that my right hand (my 'bad' hand) would rapidly tire. However, I have found that once the left hand gets going, the right one joins in and moves much faster than I would have expected.

And what about my spectacular achievements in getting off the floor and out of the bath? I am sure that an expert on muscular activity could explain to me why I can get up fairly nimbly from all fours whereas I have difficulty in raising myself from a lying or sitting position. But in the absence of such expert advice I will continue telling myself what Parkinson's has shown me; just because I can't do simple things, it is very important for me not to assume that I can't do complex ones, as I am likely to be wrong.

Whilst I am on the subject, it also seems important that other people don't make the same logical mistake as myself and assume that because some people can't do some, apparently simple actions, they are also incapable of carrying out higher order, complex tasks. Therein lies prejudice; judging people on limited information and biased assumptions.

In fact, with Parkinson's, assumptions are a waste of time. Imagination is what is needed and is what works.

7
DRUGS

Considering my past lack of experience with drugs, albeit 'recreational' ones, I have certainly made up for it since developing Parkinson's Disease.

The drug that I have found invaluable in helping my symptoms of Parkinson's is levodopa, which I currently take in the form of 'Sinemet Plus', its trade name. However, it was several years before I started to take levodopa and I had significant problems with it when I first did so. It took me about seven months to acclimatise to the drug. Levodopa is now very helpful to me, but I am aware that I am likely to require larger doses in the future and that, at some point, unless I am very lucky, I shall start experiencing dyskinesias: involuntary movements which can resemble writhing or sudden physical jerks, as a result of taking the drug. (Incidentally, since writing this, I was told by a consultant that the latest thinking on the subject suggests that levodopa may not cause the writhing movements and so there is no longer a need for such caution in taking the drug. My initial euphoric response was dampened, however, when the consultant followed up by explaining that the current thinking is that one will develop the dyskinesias anyway, levodopa or no levodopa!)

When I first started to take levodopa I understandably did so before or with meals. I had no contrary advice. My reaction was fast and intense. I would feel very hot, would sweat profusely, would feel faint and could not continue eating the meal. Although I had started on a low dosage of the drug, this was further decreased to try to improve matters, but the above reactions continued although with less force. I had to be careful to arrange my work so that the side effects had worn off before I had any tasks to do. Then I read information about nutrition and Parkinson's, which suggested that some people find it physically upsetting to eat protein at the same time as taking levodopa. Apparently, both protein and levodopa compete to cross the blood-brain barrier and so I surmised that I could be feeling the repercussions of their competition. I also read that some people find it more beneficial to take levodopa on an empty stomach and some benefit from postponing their intake of protein until late in the day. So, I decided to give the levodopa a fighting chance to get through that blood brain barrier with as little trouble as possible. I didn't much like the idea of being a battle-ground. I tried various permutations on the themes of protein and levodopa and over the next seven months the battleground changed into a peaceful pastureland.

First of all, I stopped taking levodopa with a protein meal during the daytime. This essentially meant that I had porridge made with soya milk and fruit for breakfast, a lunch consisting of vegetable soup and a bread roll (no butter) with tomato or lettuce and my main meal in the evening. I took the levodopa at least an hour and a quarter before each meal, apart from late in the evening when I took the tablet just before going to bed. I rapidly felt better and was able to increase my levodopa intake to what it was supposed to be. Unusual symptoms developed, however! After taking a levodopa tablet there was approximately twenty minutes of calm. Then I would burp a few times. After that I would sweat for about ten minutes. Finally, I would fall asleep for about twenty minutes, interrupted by one or two loud snorts This brought me to approximately an hour post levodopa intake and at last I began to gain benefits from the drug: I could write fairly successfully; I could stand up straight without stooping; I had a lot more energy; all sorts of aches and pains in my right arm would go away. And at that time these benefits lasted for about four hours.

I was delighted. This was the most improvement I had experienced since first developing Parkinson's. I started to look forward to taking the tablets. I had three tablets per day. I would take the first one of the day well over an hour before I had to get up. Then I had time to go through the burping, sweating, sleeping and snorting routine before having to face the day. At lunchtime I also made sure that I had over an hour in which to burp, sweat, sleep and snort before greeting the afternoon. In the evening I was able to wait to take the necessary tablet until going to bed and this time the pattern stopped at the sleeping part. I slept wonderfully.

When I had been taking dopamine successfully for one year my regime increased to four tablets each day. The first one was at about six in the morning. I would get up at about eight thirty, have a fairly protein-free breakfast (cereal and fruit) at around nine-thirty and would have my second tablet of the day at about noon. This tablet worked extremely well if I hadn't eaten any more than I have described. The slight hunger I felt was well worth being able to stand (fairly) straight, being able to write and shaking far less, let alone being able to hold items and generally having more energy. However, if I had snacked and particularly if this involved protein, then I felt very little benefit at all.

My third tablet of the day came at about five pm. In the meantime, I would have eaten some bread and salad at around two thirty pm, giving myself at least two hours before the third tablet. I then ate whatever I wanted, including protein, at around seven pm. I also drank a glass of wine if I wanted to.

As I write this, it is two years since I started to take levodopa and I currently take five tablets per day. The general principles are the same as before, including the avoidance of protein in the daytime, and my tablet times are approximately 7am, 11am, 3pm, 7pm and 11pm.

I take my last tablet of the day as I am undressing for bed. As I have already mentioned, I am slow at undressing and so my tablet has time to take action by the time I have read a little in bed and have gone to sleep. As I have also mentioned I sleep very well since taking levodopa.

On re-reading this chapter I realise that it will be mind-numbingly boring for most people. Very few people will be interested in my intake of food and tablets. That is not surprising. However, the point of my account is to stress the importance of monitoring and recording the effects on one's behaviour of these powerful brain-altering drugs, particularly if one is having any problem with them. It may be that simple adjustments, such as I have mentioned, could improve matters.

Since I was first diagnosed with Parkinson's I have been prescribed numerous drugs by consultants and their assistants. At first I took them without question, but as I began to realise that they had all manner of possible side effects I decided that I should make informed choices before taking these drugs and also that I should monitor their effects on me. After all, the doctors cannot possibly predict exactly the impact which each drug will have on each different individual. The side effects of these drugs can be significant and wide-ranging. They can affect the digestive system, the urinary system, the skin, the heart and the nervous system amongst other possibilities. I remember reading 'dark saliva' as being a side effect of one drug and finding this quite unimaginable until my pillowslip became stained. I now manage this side effect by changing my pillowslip every day.

The first drug I was prescribed, soon after being diagnosed with Parkinson's, was a dopamine agonist and I was advised to take it initially in very small doses, accompanied by an anti-sickness drug. I didn't feel sick and soon the amount of drug was increased. I remember being nervous about the side effects I had been warned of, including possible hallucinations. I imagined suddenly seeing the equivalent of Banquo's ghost, turning up at professional meetings. Luckily, no hallucinations manifested themselves. However, I did experience a lot of sleepiness during the daytime and this was difficult to manage, particularly as the Parkinson's symptoms did not seem to show any signs of improvement. It felt as though the medication was adding to my problems, rather than giving me any help. I had to find all kinds of methods of keeping myself awake, particularly when using a computer. (I began to think that computers, in conjunction with the dopamine agonist, had some kind of influence over the sleep patterns of the brain.) I regularly reported the state of affairs to my hospital consultant who basically did nothing about it and kept prescribing the same drug. I can't believe that I put up with this situation for nearly five years, but I did! I thought I had no alternative. Eventually, I was finding the sleepiness so stressful that I rebelled, decreased my dosage and eventually came off the drug altogether. I decided at that point to start taking levodopa instead. If I had the opportunity to live this time over again I would complain far more vociferously in the first place and would not accept so readily that nothing could be done to help me.

Anti-Parkinson's drugs may affect behaviour in ways that can be disturbing for the individual, particularly if they do not realise that their behaviour is linked to a drug they are taking. In recent years there have been a growing number of stories in the media about people who have developed an obsession with gambling as a result of taking anti-Parkinson's drugs, particularly dopamine agonists. Some people have developed a compulsion to gamble away their money and this has obviously had a harmful effect on their lives. It seems that some individuals show obsessional behaviour when they take dopamine agonists or levodopa and that this can manifest itself in different ways, including gambling. This is a powerful illustration of how much our behaviour can be influenced by our chemical make-up.

My experience of a dopamine agonist was different but similar. Little did I know that my psychiatrist colleague had got it right when I first declared that I had Parkinson's. He rang me to sympathise but very soon asked me what my sex-drive was like. At first I thought he was joking and I gave him a predictable non-answer. But he was being serious. He told me that it was known that people with Parkinson's sometimes developed a stronger sex-drive as a result of some of the drugs they were given. I didn't take a lot of notice of what he'd said but every so often it would come back to me and on one occasion I asked the hospital consultant's assistant about the issue. I said that I'd heard that some Parkinson's drugs increased one's sex-drive and I wondered which they were. 'You're on one,' he said.

So, I tried to investigate further the side effects of dopamine agonists and found a tiny bit of information stating that, in a very small number of cases, these drugs could affect a person's sex-drive. But the effect was generally described as decreasing, not increasing, the drive. I then forgot about the issue.

I don't want to embarrass myself, my family, friends and colleagues by going into details, but after a couple of years of taking the drug I discovered that I was among the supposedly very small number of cases mentioned above and that the change in me was exponentially towards the increase. Luckily, my newly found ardour was all directed towards my husband who now looks back at his time of living with a femme fatale with amused nostalgia. I was lucky, but I am sure that someone without an understanding partner, or with no partner at all, could have been quite worried about this marked, obsessive, change in his or her behaviour. I have recently noticed that there has been an increase in general information and research about the effect of anti-Parkinson's drugs on sexual behaviour and that is all to the good.

My experience of brain-altering drugs has given me a healthy respect for them. After all, I am currently on a drug that can alter my handwriting in a period of just over an hour. I find that amazing. Whatever drug is now prescribed for me, I look up its possible side effects in books and journals, as well as on the internet and then I make a decision as to whether I shall take it or not. I discuss this with my doctor who is very supportive. In fact, I have found most medical people supportive. The only lack of support I experienced came from the individual mentioned above, who simply did not take notice when I regularly complained of sleepiness.

Just as it is important for a person with Parkinson's to understand the effects of the drugs they take, so it is equally important for them to take the drugs at the correct times. Such powerful medication cannot be taken haphazardly. So it is sad that hospitals sometimes seem oblivious to this fact. I went into hospital for a minor operation a while ago and kept my daily dose of Parkinson's drugs with me. For this, I was roundly told off by the pharmacist who expressly came on the ward to do so, loudly. Eventually, my consultant apologised for the pharmacist's behaviour and agreed to review the situation as regards Parkinson's sufferers who attended the hospital. This was necessary in view of the intensely individual need to take the drugs at particular times and not at times which happen to be convenient for the hospital. More recently the Parkinson's Disease Society has been working to achieve this aim, using a campaign called, 'Get it on time'.

8
ALL CHANGE

What I have written so far just about takes me to the time when I had had Parkinson's for approximately eight years, although the diagnosis was around six years old. I had continued to work full-time and had very much enjoyed doing so, but recently I had started to notice an increase in my symptoms.

I was finding it difficult to get going in the mornings. I was getting slower at washing and dressing and a nine o'clock work start, particularly if it involved much travelling to the place of work, was proving more difficult. Climbing up and down stairs, walking down corridors, opening doors, carrying cumbersome bags, opening test cases, carrying books, tidying piles of paper, all were becoming an effort, to the extent that they were becoming stressful. Sometimes I felt unsteady on my feet, occasionally veering without warning so that I would bump into door openings and lurch towards people. My shaking was increasing at times although at other times I hardly shook at all. The unpredictability of the symptoms was stressful in itself because it was difficult to prepare for the day, not knowing how I would feel when giving a talk or conducting an interview. Nevertheless, I was giving a lot of supervision sessions and did not find these difficult, partly because they involved very limited movement and partly because my supervision consulting room was very close to home.

Also, I was compiling and typing numerous reports on the computer but, again, did not find this to be an arduous task.

So I was in a bit of a quandary. On the one hand I was very much enjoying my work, but on the other I was finding it increasingly tiring to get to work and to carry out the movements I needed in order to work. Colleagues were very encouraging, reminding me that other people could carry my bags and open doors for me, whereas it was harder to find people to give lectures, assess people who had special educational needs and compile reports. My husband was extremely helpful, driving me to my places of work and picking me up when I had finished. Although I could still drive I had decided to take up his offer of lifts, to conserve my energy. My youngest son, who was temporarily living with us, took over the cooking and I was very grateful for that. Nevertheless, despite all this help I became steadily more tired after very little effort and I became increasingly more aware that Parkinson's is very much a disorder of movement, particularly when one is trying to initiate movements. At times, when I became tired I would also become very cold and had to sit still and warm up, in order to recuperate. Each time my levodopa tablet wore off I was experiencing a noticeable deterioration in my symptoms, which would then improve again when the next tablet started working. I had come to a crossroads. What should I do about work? On the one hand I enjoyed it; I did not want to let people down and felt that a little more effort would keep me going. On the other hand the exhaustion was significant and there was little energy left over for anything but work. I was becoming irritable at times at the suggestion of socialising because I was so tired.

Then the question arose about temporarily living in France. My youngest son needed somewhere to live for a year, to do some extra studies and there was not enough room for all three of us in our London flat. Neither could we afford to rent another flat for him and pay all the accompanying bills. However, we had recently acquired a small place in France. If Jack and I went to live in France for a year this would free up the flat in England and all three of us would be housed. Obviously, I would have to stop working for the year, apart from the possibility of some work over the Internet. But this would give us the opportunity to think over the work situation, to practise living on pensions and to make longer-term plans. Jack thought it was a good idea. As for me, I had wanted to spend some time in France for a while. My mother was French; I had spent two years at school in Paris as a child and when I had left I had spoken French fluently. However, this was many years ago; new ways of living such as computer technology had given rise to new forms of language and during that time my French had deteriorated. For a long time I had wanted to return to France to brush it up. But the major reason for considering moving to France for a year was the Parkinson's reason. My Parkinson's was enthusiastically increasing by leaps and bounds and was leaving me behind. I needed an opportunity to readjust, to catch up with its pace. It was not the first time that Parkinson's had brought major change into my life.

So, after a good six months of considerations, preparations, transitions and good-byes, we were on our way to Dover in a very full car which contained, amongst other things, several months' supply of Parkinson's drugs. Only a year prior to this I would not have thought I would have made the decisions that had led to this journey. Two years before, it would have been unbelievable. At that time I had had some thought in mind that I would work for at least another five years. Three years back and I was still very much enjoying the variety and excitement of working in schools, colleges and nurseries, with children, young people, families and all manner of staff, to see if we could make a difference in difficult situations by working together. Some of the situations were complex and wearing, but they were always interesting, stimulating and invariably inspired hope about human nature; someone always emerged from these situations as having the creativity to imagine change and the determination to do what it took to carry it through. A sense of humour always helped of course, as well as an ability to accept less than perfect outcomes.

And now I had to contemplate my own change and to hope that I could develop the imagination necessary to carry it through. I also suspected that a lot of humour would be necessary, particularly when trying to tolerate the imperfect.

As we travelled South, through France, I wondered how

my Parkinson's would affect my French. I had recently been aware that, particularly at times when I was self-conscious, my words had developed a tendency to peter out in English; what would they do in French? Another thing I had noticed was that my voice had become quieter. At least, it was not actually me who had noticed; other people had pointed it out to me and my consultant had referred me to a speech therapist, who had taped my voice and played it back to me. This was very useful because until then I had not realised how quiet I sounded and I resolved to make an effort to speak louder. Apparently it is quite usual for Parkinson's sufferers to have these sorts of problems with speech and language and I wondered if I would have a major problem when speaking French. My husband didn't speak French, although he wanted me to teach him, and so I would be the main communicator and negotiator to start with. We would have to negotiate with our French bank, with French Telecom, with the car registration people, with a tax office, with the local mayor and no doubt with many other officials. How would French officialdom take to a shaking English woman? I would not be able to hide away to conceal my embarrassment. I started rehearsing, 'J'ai une maladie de Parkinson', to explain myself if the occasion called for it.

We took three days travelling to the South West of France and arrived with the heat. The Pyrenees were not visible as they would be in the colder weather and when rain was forecast. Our small house was in an isolated spot, on the edge of a hamlet and five kilometres from the nearest village. We would value this isolation but not on the first night.

Jack woke me up at two in the morning to tell me that he had heard two or three men outside on the balcony talking, but he had not been able to understand what they were saying. He had put on the outside lights, hoping that this would encourage them to depart, but they were still there. I listened and could hear them talking, but could not make out their words. Then they moved off the balcony and started circling the house. After some whispered discussion we decided that we had better call the 'Gendarmerie' and dialled 17, the French equivalent of 999. The gendarmes arrived within half an hour; pretty good going when we realised how far they had had to drive. They banged on the front door and we gratefully opened up to three large men in uniform with truncheons and guns, carrying powerful torches. We all looked round the outside of the house, but the intruders had gone. The police were extremely reassuring and very solicitous towards me, emphasising several times that we had done the right thing and that we should do so again if the same circumstances arose. It was only after they had gone that I realised I had not explained my shaking. I had totally forgotten my prepared French sentence about my 'maladie de Parkinson'. The police must have thought that I had been in a particularly bad state of nerves as a result of our experience! Just to reassure the faint-hearted, we never again experienced any repetition of the event during all the time we spent in France. Neither did we discover who had been wandering around that night.

9
TIME AND MOTION
(and some frustration)

One of the major characteristics of Parkinson's is slowness of movement and for me that means that everything takes me much more time than it used to take. That wouldn't matter if other people had also slowed down, but they haven't. So there is a mismatch between my expectation of how fast I can move and other people's expectations of how fast I am able to move, unless they understand Parkinson's. This mismatch can cause me to feel embarrassed, as when an eager secretary says, 'follow me' and then discovers that she has lost me; I am still slowly trundling behind, a corridor away. By the time I left England this kind of thing was happening to me more and more frequently.

However, very soon after coming to France I realised that I now had all the time I needed to carry out ordinary physical activities and that at last I was not holding anyone up by doing so. We were in a situation where we had very few day-to-day obligations. It didn't matter if I took over an hour to get dressed in the morning and all day to prepare supper. If I became tired I could sit down and read or look at the view. I had the luxury of having enough time. More than that, I had the opportunity to find out how much time I really needed to carry out various activities. I could establish my own baseline. Recently, before coming to France, I hadn't been sure if I was further slowing down or whether I was just generally tired out and needed some rest and leisure to put me back at what I had come to accept as my state of equilibrium.

I rapidly established that my baseline was now very different from those of most of the population and that it differed from mine, less than a year prior to coming to France. What now took me an hour probably took other people a quarter of the time. Physically, I had become a different person from the one I was a year ago. I seemed to have entered a new phase of Parkinson's.

This realisation took some time for me to accept, probably because I didn't want to accept it. I felt sad at what I had lost and I was also frightened. Until then I felt that I had managed my Parkinson's, but now it was managing me. I suppose that anyone who has a deteriorating condition measures their current capabilities in terms of what they used to do. Perhaps if my job had been more sedentary; for example, composing crossword puzzles or being a television film critic, then I would not have noticed quite so much change in myself. (Incidentally, I realise that I am not doing justice to these two occupations!) But my career had entailed a fair amount of physical energy, both in moving around a lot and in terms of enthusing and motivating people. I missed this aspect of my work. Sometimes at night I would dream about working with staff and colleagues in schools and other institutions. I remembered some of the funny and challenging situations that had happened. I told someone how much I missed working with families and I felt very angry when they suggested that, as an alternative, I might consider doing voluntary work with children. If I had the energy to do voluntary work, I complained to myself, then I wouldn't have a problem. How could this person be so obtuse?

In short, I was feeling angry about having Parkinson's. I realised that I had deteriorated physically and was alarmed about it.

Looking back and trying to take stock in retrospect, I can see that my problems were not only that my symptoms were increasing, but also that I was finding it hard, physically and psychologically, to deal with the 'on-off', stop-go results of taking levodopa.

Professionals talk about the 'on-off' effect which levodopa can exert on those who take it. Basically this means that when the drug is working (the 'on' phase) and presumably making up for some of the missing dopamine, one feels comparatively normal. In my case the most striking effect I notice is being able to stand up straight with no need to stoop. I also have far more energy and both of these effects immediately give me a feeling of wellbeing. Then there is the fact that I shake less and for a short while my writing is readable. All my fine motor skills function better. For me, the results of all these improvements are optimism and positivity. I feel that I can tackle all those little jobs that seemed daunting. I enjoy being out shopping, being round at friends', being out in a restaurant, doing every day tasks. I feel able to take on commitments. I can even feel hopeful that the Parkinson's is over; that it was all a dream. This 'on' period lasts for an hour or two at the most. Then the 'off' period starts. From one minute to the next I can no longer do the things that I engaged in just a short while ago. Now I feel very tired if I tackle a task such as peeling a potato; my back muscles hurt; my right arm tightens up painfully; I can't write legibly; I stoop; my legs buckle; I drop things; I can become very cold. I feel as though I had aged twenty years in ten minutes. My feeling of optimism is not so much lost as drowned in exhaustion. Luckily, within another hour or two I will be able to take another dose of levodopa but, to add to the above confusion I cannot assume that the next dose will always have the same positive effect as the last one. At least once per day the drug has very little effect at all; for example, as I have already described, I find that it works far less well if I have recently eaten protein. There are also times when it does not seem to work for no reason I can fathom. So one is living in a very unpredictable world, in my case bounded by one to two hour intervals. Basically, the routine is two hours 'on' followed by two hours 'off', with some unpredictable hours as well. At first, when one experiences the 'on' sensations, there is a tendency to feel that one is back to normal because so much of what used to be normal has returned. Then the 'off' period begins and hope sinks.

If one considers the 'on-off' phenomenon, one sees that it attacks a person's sense of continuity. Healthy people tend to assume that how they were physically feeling a few minutes ago, a few hours ago and even a few days ago is how they expect to feel now. Without that sense of continuity it is very hard to plan sensibly for the short term, let alone the long term. I do not think that it is an overstatement to say that a sense of continuity supports one's sense of self: one's sense of who one is. Being human demands that we take some things for granted. One can't literally live in the present. It is natural to predict the immediate future from the present and the immediate past. When one's bodily sensations frequently change it is hard to guess how one will be feeling in a few hours' time, let alone tomorrow. Hence, there is a danger of assuming that one has lost control and that there is no point in planning any more.

It is hard for other people too. They see that their friend or relation can do something one day and so they naturally assume that the person can do the same thing the next day. If the person cannot, then in some people there must be a lurking doubt about malingering! It is natural to assume that people can or can't do things, not that they are able to do the thing one minute, but not the next. People are used to expecting continuity from others just as they expect it in themselves. We are all creatures of habit. Many of the reassuring remarks made by other people (such as: 'you don't look any different to me'; 'I haven't noticed any change in you'; 'I know how you feel; I've felt like that since I've got older') are said to reassure the persons making and receiving the remarks that things are still as they were. Unfortunately, however, the truth is that things have changed and in my case these remarks don't reassure me at all. All they do is suggest to me that perhaps I sound as though I'm exaggerating my difficulties. Perhaps the only way to explain what it is like to others is by using similes; for me the 'off' period is like being a car, which has run out of petrol. There is little point in saying of the car, 'It looks as though it should be able to move'. Or, saying about a string puppet whose strings have been cut, 'She looks as though she could work quite well.' The car needs petrol, the puppet needs its strings to be mended and I need dopamine. It's as simple as that.

The unpredictability with which I was living made me feel very different from others. For a while I felt like avoiding people, partly out of embarrassment but also because of a reluctance to keep explaining how I felt, in the face of other people's understandable lack of understanding of the condition.

10
A WAY FORWARD

So for a while, I felt confused and unhappy. Then came decision-making time. As I have described, I had come to a situation in which I was finding it hard to predict how well I would feel, almost from hour to hour. This was not compatible with fulfilling the responsibilities of working as a psychologist, including keeping up to date by means of regular professional training and receiving supervision. I had no choice but to decide that the official 'work' phase in my life was definitely over and to wait to see what new phase might emerge.

We returned to England for Christmas and I was offered several pieces of work but kept to my decision not to accept them. It had been hard enough to make this decision and I did not wish to repeat the process. Nevertheless, I felt somewhat jealous of two ex-colleagues, both retired from their long-term careers as psychologists, but who were both engaged in psychological projects, which they evidently found very fulfilling. 'That's the sort of thing I had wanted to do', I thought.

But then I slowly started to become aware of things I enjoyed, or thought I might enjoy, now that I was no longer officially working as a psychologist. One was writing: I had written at least half of a novel a few years back but had abandoned it, owing to a lack of time. There were also other areas of writing, which interested me; one being to write about the experience of having Parkinson's. I was also keen on continuing to improve my French, which had already benefited from being practised in France for several months and from my regular reading in French. There was also other reading which interested me, especially in the area of Psychology. And then, (I felt particularly reluctant to admit this to myself at first), and then, there was cooking!

I had never been a good cook. Before I developed Parkinson's I had spent much of my life studying or working, as well as bringing up a family and I did not have time to cook, other than very basic meals. I reasoned that people would always find themselves something out of the ordinary to eat if they wanted it, but they were less likely to do the cleaning. So, until I could pay for help, I cleaned the toilet, and the bathroom, and the kitchen, and other rooms, together with other household tasks, such as monumental amounts of tidying and organising, and left the task of cooking to the experts. The most successful experts were my three sons, all of who have turned out to be masters of the art of cookery. My first son started to order a magazine called 'Cordon Bleu' at the age of nine and this would rapidly disappear into his bedroom after landing on our doormat. He has since told me that he used to daydream in lessons at school about the meal he would concoct that night. When my second son reached the age of nine he asked if he could have his portion of the house-keeping money so that he could plan and cook his own dishes and he did so for over year. Later on this son worked for a while as a chef. My third son was older when he turned to cookery but at around twenty-one years old he ran a chalet in the Alps and cooked, daily, for sixteen people, for five months. (For those who feel alarmed at this account of neglected sons I can assure them that all three have developed into well-adjusted adults who eat healthily!)

However, as for me, I had not been successful in the art of cuisine. A friend of ours who came round to dinner with his wife was heard to sigh with relief when I apologised for having bought a ready cooked supper from Waitrose for the meal, rather than having served up home cooking!

I was surprised when I realised how interested I was in learning to cook successfully and friends and relatives were even more surprised. But it made sense when I thought about the entertaining part. Being able to cook facilitates hospitality. I have always enjoyed communicating with people. That was one of the reasons for my choice of career in the first place. My temporary avoidance of social company, which I have described above, was out of character. Cooking and entertaining fitted in easily with what I felt was meaningful in life. And then of course there was the possibility that, as my Parkinson's developed, I would find it harder to go out and so it made sense to invite people over to our place.

However, achievement of this cookery aim would not be without its difficulties: I have explained that my fine motor control was one of my biggest problems; not only was that so, but I rapidly became exhausted when peeling, chopping, and cutting, let alone when mixing or trying to roll pastry. I would have to find ways around these difficulties; I knew that there were mechanical devices available to help with the chopping and mixing and no doubt with other (to me) esoteric cookery skills and I resolved to get to know them.

After all, I reasoned to myself, I had faced other apparently insurmountable learning situations in life, such as taking Physics, Chemistry and Zoology A levels in my early twenties, as a young mother. This had been particularly challenging because I had not studied sciences at all before this time, my meandering school career having led me through English, French and History A levels, for no sensible reason except that they were the subjects available at the umpteenth school I was attending at the time. So, for a long time I had known that just because you have never been able to do something in the past, it doesn't necessarily mean that you won't be able to do it in the future. And of course, there was the important lesson I had learned from Parkinson's: to look for ways around problematic situations. Not that creative use of one's environment is the prerogative of Parkinson's. For example, when I was studying those A levels in my early twenties, with two young children to look after, I bought a playpen and put myself inside the pen, with my books and papers, whilst the children had the run of the room.

By the time we returned to France, after Christmas, I was daring to think that my future might possibly look meaningful again and above all that it contained the possibility of new experiences. I felt more hopeful now that I was focusing on what I might be able to do, rather than dwelling on what I could no longer do.

11
MOVEMENT

Parkinson's can be described medically as a movement disorder and as my Parkinson's has developed I have found that the most marked changes I have experienced have been in my movements. Other people would probably say that my shaking is the most pronounced feature of my Parkinson's but, to me, the problems I have in moving give credence to the description of Parkinson's as a disability.

I can divide my movements into two types: gross motor and fine motor (in other words, large movements and small, fiddly movements) and, as I have already described, I have far more problems with the latter than the former. I also seem to have a problem with my spatial perception and this accentuates my poor motor skills. For example, when placing an object such as a cup on a table, I tend to place it far too near the edge of the table, so that part of it overhangs the table and people around me become anxious, often reaching across and moving the cup to a safer position. Also, I have recently become aware that I must take care not to lose my balance. At the time of writing this I have only fallen once, when walking up some unfamiliar stairs, but I am very conscious that falling over is an ever-present danger in Parkinson's and so I am especially careful to do things at my pace and not, misguidedly, to attempt to adapt to someone else's pace. As with all my Parkinson's symptoms, however, the effects I've just described depend on how recently I have taken a levodopa tablet and whether it is working well or not.

My doctor told me, when I was first diagnosed, that one of the main problems in Parkinson's is in initiating movement. One symptom which doesn't trouble me much at present, but which some people with Parkinson's can suffer from severely, is 'freezing'. This is a problem with initiating movement. For example, the person wants to walk forward, possibly through a doorway, but they simply cannot move. This is not because of any intrinsic problem with their walking, since once they have started walking, it can be difficult for them to stop doing so. Hence, they may need help to start walking and to stop walking.

I have not experienced any problems in initiating my walking. I may swerve at times and as I've described, I can lose my balance, but I have not yet ever felt that I cannot walk. However, I do have problems with initiating some movements. For example, I find it hard to get out of an armchair and in such a case I can get to a point when I simply cannot move. For some reason this makes me laugh! I don't feel as though I am paralysed, instead, it feels as though I have forgotten how to get up, rather than that I am physically incapable of doing so. Previously, I described how I get up quite easily from being on all fours. So, if I get into a situation where I can't get out of the chair in the normal way, I change to my all fours manner. Incidentally, trying to get out of a chair is much harder for me if I have anything in my hand, even a little piece of paper.

I have also experienced a problem with my right hand and arm in initiating movement. For example, I might want to grasp a fork, but somehow my hand seems reluctant to carry out the movement and it would be very easy for me to go into a state of suspended animation whilst waiting for it to do so. When I've encouraged my hand to do what I want it to (by telling it to move) it is reluctant to let go of the fork. This reluctance to let go applies to my right arm too. I might be holding a door open and then I will walk on, but my arm stays with the door! At those times, people who know me very well will give my arm a little nudge to encourage it on its way. Again, for some reason this makes me laugh. I think that this may be due to my awareness of the incongruity of the situation; the fact that I need a little push to keep me going, rather like one of those old clockwork trains with which children played, when I was young.

Putting on cardigans, jackets and coats has become much more difficult. I think that my poor spatial perception adds to the problem in these cases: once I have struggled into the first sleeve, I cannot imagine the position of the entrance to the second sleeve and so cannot manoeuvre my second arm into it. It helps if I look into a full-length mirror whilst doing so, but of even greater help is having two full-length mirrors, appropriately angled so that I can see my back view as well as the front.

Turning over in bed can be problematic. I think this is because I am trying to get my back muscles to move, as when I'm getting out of a chair.

As far as my fine motor movements go, I have had

problems with them for longer than the gross motor movements and they have steadily become more difficult to carry out. My right arm and hand often feel more like a broom handle than the sensitive instruments they are supposed to be. I think that my problems with fine motor skills have five main causes:

1) only being able to perform one fine motor movement successfully, at a time;

2) a problem with initiating the movement;

3) a pronounced weakness in my right hand and a little weakness in the left hand;

4) a problem with spatially imagining the movement; and

5) shaking.

Take, for example, a situation when I am in the street: my mobile phone rings in my handbag and I want to get it out of the bag to see who is ringing or texting me. First, I need to un-zip my bag. I have to stop walking to do this because I simply cannot walk and at the same time perform a fine motor task which requires any dexterity. So I stop, possibly in a shop doorway, and try to un-zip the bag. My hand is reluctant to move to the zip and so I encourage it by telling it to do so (in my mind). I cannot mentally visualise the zip as well as I did in the past so I have to look at it to see what I am doing. This means that I have to steady the handbag with my other hand. This concentration of both hands on the task causes the right one to shake more than it has been doing and the left one to start shaking in sympathy. Let us assume that I have managed to open the zip. I now need to get the mobile out of the bag. Again, I have problems in locating the mobile in the bag because of my poor visual imagination. Then, when I have located it, I need to pull it out and my hand is reluctant to do this and feels weak. Once I have managed to remove the mobile from the bag, I need to use my fingers to press the correct keys to answer the phone or retrieve the message. Shaking makes this difficult, particularly as I tend to press the same keys two or three times! Needless to say, I hardly ever reach the phone in time to answer it and usually have to ring back.

It all sounds a bit complicated when I describe answering the mobile phone in this much detail, but I have found that the only way I can cope with fine motor tasks is to describe them in detail, break them down into small entities, practise them and try to keep relaxed. As with other areas of Parkinson's, I have found that relaxation is extremely beneficial and is a loyal friend to engage when it seems that my movements are falling apart. When things get to this stage the way forward for me is to sit as still as possible and relax. If matters do not improve, having a nap is helpful.

There is one more variable, which I have to take into account when describing the effect of Parkinson's on my fine movements and that is the repetition factor. If I have a problem with a fine motor task and keep repeating it, the movement deteriorates rapidly. So, as with so many other aspects of Parkinson's, it is important for me to recognise when to give up and think of another way around the situation. Parkinson's certainly encourages creativity!

12
EXERCISE

I have found the whole area of exercise and Parkinson's to be quite confusing. Basically, I have found that I have two opposing sets of needs as regards exercise. One is to keep mobile and active and the other is to conserve my energy, trying to avoid becoming exhausted. It has been important to keep these two factors in balance.

When I first developed Parkinson's, even before it had been diagnosed, I turned to exercise in order to try to help myself. When I didn't know I had Parkinson's and assumed that my shaking was because of stress, I decided that living a healthier life-style could only be beneficial. I joined a gym for the first time in my life, gave up coffee and practised relaxation. As regards the extra exercise I was taking, I vaguely assumed that it would increase my overall strength and that the chemicals released in my brain during exercise would be beneficial in encouraging me to relax. However, my symptoms did not improve although I did feel more relaxed and this generally made life easier to manage. Then I received the diagnosis of Parkinson's. I felt this warranted a new look at my fitness schedule and I decided to find a new gym (mine was small and had become over-crowded) where I could look for a personal trainer.

Having a personal trainer would not have occurred to me, had I not been diagnosed with Parkinson's, but I now felt that I needed professional guidance in the whole area of exercise. Jack and I found a new gym, which was spacious and welcoming. There were various trainers around and I approached one of them, Jill, who was very friendly, to ask her how to go about arranging to have a personal trainer. I also told her that I had Parkinson's. So started a relationship, which has now lasted several years and has only been interrupted by my travels to France. Jill and I have met weekly or fortnightly over the period of time and I cannot express how much this has meant to my self-esteem. Jill is much younger than me, positive, glowing with health and vitality, slim, very attractive, excellent at every exercise under the sun, intelligent and...patient. I have valued the last of these attributes above all the rest. She had not worked with anyone who had Parkinson's before she met with me, but immediately grasped the important issues such as my ability to do something one week and not the next and my increasing tendency to become suddenly exhausted.

The wonderful thing about having regular personal training input is the privilege of regularly being the focus of someone else's professional attention. In that sense it is a bit like receiving counselling, although counselling focuses on feelings and thoughts whereas Jill has focused on what I can do with my body. Having said that, I can think of many times when I have lost heart, lost confidence and Jill has encouraged me to think positively about my physical achievements, sending me off feeling proud of myself rather than being tearfully self-critical about what

I cannot do physically. The fact of seeing Jill regularly and using the sessions to review and plan, as well as for exercising, has maintained a freshness in my work with her and a sense that I keep being given a 'new start'.

I always start my sessions with Jill on the treadmill. A while ago, I was able to extend these sessions by gradually raising my speed and lengthening the time on the treadmill, but now I am aware that if I concentrate too much on improvement I may exhaust myself and have to curtail the session. So, instead I focus on maintaining my time and speed; if there is an improvement, so much the better. Occasionally, I cannot reach my usual level and so I stop. As has already been mentioned several times, however, my performance does depend on how the medication is working at the time.

When I am in France I do not have access to a treadmill and instead I start every day by bouncing on the trampette! This is a mini trampoline on which one can walk on the spot, jump and bounce. My bouncing is done each morning, facing the Pyrenees. I have a wonderful view and luckily the area is sparsely inhabited so I don't have to worry about the view I am providing. My bouncing is carried out on a veranda and so rain and snow have not stopped me, although high winds have occasionally been a problem. The work on the treadmill and the trampette, as well as work on the rower in the gym, comes under the heading of 'cardiovascular exercise'. As the name implies, the aim is to exercise the heart and lungs; very important for me I would think, now that I have considerably slowed down because of Parkinson's.

The second main area of exercise has concentrated on my general posture, balance and stability. It can be as simple as going for a walk or I can follow gentle exercises, which Jill has designed for me and has illustrated in an exercise book using stick men. I find that if I don't have this kind of practice almost every day, particularly at the beginning of the day, I tend to feel unsteady on my feet and generally shaky all over. I also stoop more, making it difficult to achieve a reasonable posture. Since coming to France I have learned more exercises, derived from yoga, from a relaxation class that was arranged by the local French Parkinson's group. I find these exercises also very helpful when I feel unsteady.

To try to describe what I mean when I say I feel unsteady or shaky all over, I tell people that it is as though I am a wooden puppet that has had some of the strings cut. In this state I cannot rely on many of my movements. Carrying out gentle exercise, whilst looking in a full-length mirror or copying someone else, helps me to regain control of my movements and they become more coordinated.

I have already mentioned my problems with spatial awareness and I first noticed them in my work with Jill. If I could not see the part of my body to which she was referring, I had a difficulty in carrying out what she was asking me to do. We tackled this by using a full-length mirror, which we both faced, or by my facing Jill and copying her movements, as though I was looking in a mirror. I have practised the latter method in France with

Jack and have found it very useful.

The third area of exercise at which I have worked is that of stretching. One symptom of Parkinson's is stiffness and in my case my right arm can become stiff, from shoulder to wrist, and this can be very painful. Also, the more my arm stiffens up, the more my right hand clenches, adding to the stiffness and appearing strange. Stretching my arm when it hurts does a lot to alleviate the pain and regular stretching, say once or twice per day, helps to prevent the arm from stiffening in the first place. To be stretched, one either needs a purpose-built machine, as in the gym, or a willing person. Jack has proved to be an excellent stretcher! He literally pulls my arm up straight or, up and slightly diagonally across my chest. He does this for about twenty seconds at a time, for two or three stretches, approximately two or three times per day. One needs some privacy to carry out these exercises, though. I have not yet had the courage to get Jack to stretch my arm when we are in a department store or even in a small shop, however stiff it is feeling!

Very recently, Jack and I have evolved a technique for 'confusing' my painful arm, or even my leg if that is hurting. What we mean by 'confusing' is the movement of the limb in all directions, with no predictable rhythm. I relax and mentally hand over responsibility for my limb to Jack. He shakes it around and eventually the limb stops hurting. I do not know the reason for why this works although I assume that the unpredictability of where the limb will move next, acts as a counterbalance to the unrelenting, tightening and contracting which usually happens to my arm and sometimes my leg when I keep still for too long.

Parkinson's is full of anomalies and I regularly have to remind myself of some of them. On the subject of exercise, one anomaly I keep rediscovering is to do with large and small movements. I can be in a situation indoors where I feel quite limited in my movement, for example: my right arm muscles may be very tight; I may be finding it hard to get up out of my chair; my walking seems unsteady and generally I feel that I am lurching around the place in a clumsy manner. In that situation I find small, fine motor movements, such as picking up the phone, very difficult. However, I can then go outside and walk with large strides, depending where I am in my medication regime. Similarly, Jack who is an artist, has encouraged me to draw and to use big, confident movements when doing so. My artistic offerings have left a lot to be desired, but at least they have reminded me that large movements are far easier for me than small ones. I only wish that I didn't keep forgetting this!

I have gradually had to decrease the intensity of exercise that I take because of the tiredness factor, but I find it invaluable to start each day with some exercise, including movements that encourage mobility. The rule I've tried to follow is that to keep mobile you have to keep moving.

13
SLEEP

I have had mainly positive experiences of sleeping during the time I have had Parkinson's. The exception to this was the first six months or so after I had been diagnosed. I hardly slept at all during this period. I am not sure whether the reason for my insomnia was psychological, a reaction to the diagnosis, or whether it was physical, an alteration in brain chemistry caused by the Parkinson's, perhaps. I have read since that many people with Parkinson's suffer from sleep disturbances.

I was reluctant to take sleeping tablets, but in the end was persuaded to do so by a consultant's assistant. She recommended amitriptyline, an anti-depressant. I stated strongly that I wasn't depressed, but she explained to me that in very small doses amitriptyline helps sleep and that larger doses are needed to combat depression. From my first night of taking the drug I slept peacefully and I was very grateful to the consultant's assistant for her advice. I carried on taking it for over a year and had no side effects. When I stopped my nightly tablet of amitriptyline there were no repercussions. I was very impressed.

After that my sleep was normal during the five years or so that I took a dopamine agonist (before I started on levodopa). When I eventually moved on to levodopa I slept better at night than I ever have in my life. In Chapter seven I described my experiences of getting used to levodopa and the effects of taking a tablet, including falling asleep. In the daytime I would wake, refreshed, after a nap of about twenty minutes, but the effect of taking a tablet at bedtime was that I remained soundly asleep during the night. When I eventually got used to taking levodopa I ceased needing to nap during the day, but continued to sleep well at night. So, although my dosage of levodopa has gradually increased and the number of tablets I take has changed, I have continued to take one levodopa at bedtime to help with my sleep.

One of the warnings given to a patient who is about to embark on the levodopa experience is that they may get hallucinations and/or very vivid dreams. I have been lucky in that I have not experienced hallucinations but my dreams have altered. I would not say that they are particularly vivid, but the change I have noticed is that I remember many dreams now, whereas I hardly ever remembered them at all in the past. It has made my sleep life more interesting! In fact I feel that I benefit far more from sleep since taking levodopa: I sleep more deeply, for longer and I enjoy dreaming. This is definitely an area of my life that has improved since having Parkinson's.

In France, quite a lot of the Parkinson's literature focuses on ways in which people may eventually be screened for Parkinson's. Research is developing which seems to indicate certain characteristics which may one day be used to predict which currently healthy people may eventually develop Parkinson's. One indicator is having disturbed sleep with waking dreams. As a child and a young person

I had waking dreams at times and now I wonder whether this was an indicator that one day I would develop Parkinson's. The other indicators are the loss of the sense of smell and fluctuations in body temperature. I certainly suffered from the latter, near to my Parkinson's diagnosis, but not the former. My sense of smell seems to be intact. However, for several years I have had the experience of smelling things which have appeared as images on the television. For example, if I see a wood fire on television I may smell the burning wood.

Two of the factors which can contribute to disturbed sleep in Parkinson's are shaking and stiffness. I have found that the levodopa tablet that I take just before going to bed helps diminish the shaking. I also practice relaxation exercises when I lie down to go to sleep and these also help the shaking. As regards the stiffness, my right arm often tenses up and becomes stiff and painful, anywhere between the shoulder and wrist. Relaxation also helps with this, as does the levodopa tablet. If the stiffness and pain do not go away, Jack helps a lot by pulling my arm. I can feel the pain draining away from my shoulder down to my wrist when my arm is stretched. There is a strange side effect though; being stretched makes me yawn!

It also helps with the stiffness if my arm is 'confused', as described in the previous chapter.

People with Parkinson's often describe a difficulty in turning over in bed. My experience of this is when I am lying on my back. I can't easily turn over to my left side although I find it less difficult when turning onto my right side. The feeling is like that which I have when trying to get up from a deep settee. It is as though I have forgotten how to do it.

A few years ago I researched the right height of bed for optimising my ability to get in and out of bed. I found that either a very high bed or a very low one was the most useful. The high bed is obviously helpful in that it is close to one's standing position. However, I have found that a *very* low bed is also useful so long as I get in and out of it on all fours!

A lady whom I have met through the local French Parkinson's group, an informal, social group that meets every six weeks, has told me that the more she sleeps the less her Parkinson's symptoms trouble her when she is awake.

I have found that having enough satisfying sleep has been indispensable to me since I have had Parkinson's. Potential exhaustion is one of the ever-present themes in this condition and, having learned that there is no point in my trying to force myself on when I am tired, I have altered my life style as regards sleeping to ensure that I optimise what energy I have got. So I get up later than I used to, I ensure that I sleep in an environment that caters for my needs and I thank whoever and whatever I should thank for my levodopa tablets!

On the relatively few occasions that I have become very depressed at having Parkinson's, these have coincided with my being over-tired, cold and possibly hungry. I have almost come to a halt as regards movement and my mood has been very low. I have learned that the only way of dealing with this situation is for me to go to bed, warm up, have a hot, sweet drink (my favourite is milk with honey and a little brandy) and sleep. The person who eventually rises from the bed is a much more positive creature!

A final observation is that Parkinson's sufferers do not shake when they are asleep. At least, I don't shake when I am asleep and I have read that this is the common experience. What I have discovered in addition is that if I daydream I don't shake either. However, the daydream has to happen spontaneously. I can't bring it on by willing it; I have to discover myself in a daydream without having been aware of the transition from conscious thought to the daydream state. Then I discover that I am not shaking. Of course, as soon as I notice I am daydreaming I start shaking again! I have thought that if only I could find a way of bringing on daydreams at will, I would be able to improve my problem with shaking. So far I have not noticed any research on this subject but would be very interested if there were.

14
COMMUNICATING

I have always enjoyed communicating with people, as proved when I was called a 'bavarde' (chatterbox) at the age of nine by my teacher at school in Paris. Mind you, I was quite proud of this criticism, indicating as it did that I had mastered the language and was no longer left out of conversations with the other children. My experience of living in France for a couple of years as a child, having French as a second language and the problems this gave me in socialising and making friends, was an important factor in the empathy I felt for the 'second language' children whom I later met as a psychologist in schools in England.

Many years after my time at school in France I became a teacher, a lecturer, a psychologist and eventually rounded off the 'speaking' part of my career by giving talks about special educational needs and some on psychology, in different parts of the country. What I particularly enjoyed about these talks was getting through to people, bringing new ideas to some and making some complex ideas accessible to others. I was particularly buoyed up when I felt that the session had been a success in terms of its being enjoyable as well as informative. An added bonus was when I was able to use humour effectively. To be honest, I was a bit of a show-off when giving talks and really enjoyed entertaining people, particularly making them laugh.

So, I found it worrying when I realised that my speech was becoming halting and unsure. This was when I had had Parkinson's for approximately nine years. At first I thought I was simply experiencing a lack of confidence and was becoming embarrassed when I was the focus of other people's attention. After all, it *is* embarrassing to be looked at by a group of people when your arms are shaking and the rest of your body appears unsteady (despite someone once telling me that my shaking had a certain relaxing, hypnotic quality about it).

Initially, I felt that self-consciousness was a sufficient explanation for my new difficulty with expressing myself. I would be in a group, say at a dinner party, and wanting to make a point as part of the discussion, would move into the conversation. But, when people gave me their attention I would do what felt like the verbal equivalent of slipping and falling over in front of them: my speech would come out more quietly than I intended; words would tumble over each other; I had to search for some words, sometimes I would speak indistinctly and, all in all, I felt that I had failed to make the point I wanted to make. Next time a break in the conversation occurred, which I would normally wish to fill, I would opt out and let someone else take the place I would have liked to occupy myself. Or, when this process had happened several times, I would sometimes summon up my determination and concentration and launch myself into the conversation with the subtlety of a speeding tank. At these times I am sure I sounded aggressive, but I didn't mean to. I was taking a desperate flying leap at the situation and using all the energy at my disposal to do so, but what I achieved in strength I lost in sensitivity. It was also difficult to be humorous because humour requires a certain lightness of touch and ease of delivery. You can't be funny when the listeners have to wait around for your next word. I felt disappointed that another ability seemed to be deteriorating.

I brought up the subject at the local Parkinson's group in France. I said that I was finding it harder to express myself in speech and wondered if anyone else was finding the same thing. People nodded and several of them stated that people with Parkinson's speak too quietly and too fast. One woman said that she had been advised to read aloud to herself in order to improve her speech and I vowed to do so myself. As I mentioned in Chapter eight, I had been encouraging myself to speak more loudly ever since a speech therapist had recorded my speaking voice and had played it back to me. I had been surprised that my voice had been so quiet. But, more recently I had become aware of the lack of clarity of some of my words and the slowness of some of my sentences. I presumed that this was a motor difficulty, caused as are other aspects of Parkinson's by the problems with muscle movement. It feels to me that it is not the words that are lacking, but the wherewithal to emit them and pronounce them. My difficulty is in translating my thoughts into speech within an acceptable time period, whereas I have no such problems when typing, for example.

One advantage of coming to France, with regard to my speech, is that I have had to concentrate on pronunciation and diction when speaking in French. I have also expanded my vocabulary and in so doing, memory does not seem to be a problem. I have particularly used the times when I have had to negotiate with officialdom to take extra care with my communication. I have found that concentrating on another language has given me more confidence when speaking English. I am now particularly aware of trying to keep my voice loud enough; the rate of my speech slow enough; my words as clear as possible and trying to keep generally relaxed when talking. The latter is to avoid shaking too much.

Talking is a major part of communication, but there are other aspects. One important one is facial expression. Early on, when I had recently been diagnosed with Parkinson's, I heard that the condition could make you lose your smile. Since then I have met several people with Parkinson's who have a fixed, impassive expression and this can make them appear sad or uninterested. When I noticed some lack of flexibility on the right side of my face I included face muscle exercises in my morning exercise routine. These involve making all the funny faces and excruciating expressions that I can dream up!

Probably the most important factor concerning communication with other people is to keep doing it, whatever difficulty there is in doing so. For me, communication keeps my friendships alive, starts new friendships, keeps me laughing and preserves my sense of perspective. Lack of communication with other people encourages me to turn inward on myself and I can become preoccupied, sad and withdrawn as a result.

I have recently started to explain (briefly!) my problem in expressing myself, if it arises, when I am with people who do not understand Parkinson's and that has helped. It is so important for me to continue communicating with people, despite the embarrassment it causes me at times. When I am genuinely communicating with someone, the fact that I have Parkinson's becomes irrelevant.

15
SOME THOUGHTS

My original aim in writing this book was to give people who had received a diagnosis of Parkinson's some idea of how the disease had affected another person - myself. Although everyone with Parkinson's has a different experience of the disease, there are some similarities and anyway, when a person has been diagnosed with a comparatively rare condition, he or she is likely to be curious to know how it has affected others.

However, whilst writing the book I have found that I have learned much that I had not realised about how Parkinson's has affected me and how I have thought and felt about it. So I have ended up not only writing for other people but for myself as well. I have also become more aware of how important it is for friends, relatives and others, such as employers, to understand what it is like to have the disease, so I have been writing for them as well.

It is no good pretending that a diagnosis of Parkinson's is welcome, unless it is an alternative to something much more serious, and I was shocked by it, no matter how brave a face I managed to get together. Furthermore, as the condition has progressed I have sometimes felt angry and upset when I have found that my independence has become increasingly curtailed. I have felt other negative emotions also, such as envy and jealousy of those who are not similarly hampered, irritation with those who seem incapable of understanding how it feels to have Parkinson's (despite my detailed and excellent descriptions!) and sometimes I have plunged into self-pity and have felt hopeless about the future.

But luckily, these feelings do not usually last long. Like all of us, I have been in difficult situations before and I have developed ways of tackling the problems which life has thrown at me. Whenever I have been in danger of being submerged by Parkinson's I have used what I have learned from problems I have had in the past and I have found that Parkinson's responds as well as any other troubles have responded. So, if I met someone who had recently been diagnosed with Parkinson's and who was worried about how they were going to deal with the situation, I would remind them that they already have the wherewithal to manage it, by using the techniques they have used in the past for coping with problems.

People's problems are varied. One can give examples such as broken relationships, unhappy childhood, abuse, bereavement, loneliness, poverty, bullying and fear. There are countless others, the severity of which are judged by our own experience. However, the important factor is to what extent and how we overcame problems in the past. What we managed in the past we can use to help us manage in the future, including as regards Parkinson's Disease. If we feel that we didn't manage in the past, now may be the time to ask for help. The ability to be able to ask another person for help is in itself a great strength.

I said early on in this book that I was surprised to have

been diagnosed with Parkinson's and that was absolutely true. Although I theoretically knew that I could contract all manner of diseases, I was used to being protected by statistics; if I had been told before I had developed Parkinson's that I would have a 2 in 100 chance of doing so, I would have assumed that I would be among the 98. I was also surprised that there was a medical condition called Parkinson's which contained under its umbrella such apparently unconnected feelings and behaviours such as: readily becoming cold; having small, deteriorating hand writing; having lost my right arm swing and having turned into someone who shook mildly most of the time and shook strongly in stressful situations. I found Parkinson's to be a very surprising condition.

Early on amongst my new feelings was one of gratitude that the medical profession took my condition so seriously. No longer was I left to manage on my own with what I had assumed was a reaction to stress. Instead, I was being offered all kinds of medication and expert advice. I was referred to a Parkinson's specialist consultant and have been offered six monthly appointments with a consultant ever since. I became aware that a vast programme of research was going on, to try to ameliorate and even cure the condition. I felt supported. I became used to having Parkinson's and for quite a while I was not particularly worried about the consequences.

It was about eight years into the disease, when exhaustion started to take hold, when I became unsteady on my feet, when cutting my food became very difficult, when I fumbled to open my purse at check-outs, when I couldn't easily get out of a chair, when dressing, undressing and washing presented significant problems, that I started to realise that Parkinson's meant business and that I could not ignore this fact for much longer. I became aware that I really did have a deteriorating condition and that there were things, such as working, which I would have to stop and other things, such as handwriting a page of notes, that I would never be able to do again.

'Never' is a scary word that is associated in my mind with giving up and ultimately death. As the Parkinson's has progressed I have sometimes felt that it has made the decision for me, and that now I am on a one-way road, downwards, 'never' becoming a reality, in slow motion. Every time I have become aware of some other ability that I am losing, I have felt that I am witnessing my own slow death, my own deconstruction. At those times I worry about the future. What will happen if I can't manage to look after myself at all? Am I becoming a burden?

However, the pendulum then swings the other way, either because of a chance occurrence or because I encourage it to do so. An example of the former is when someone asks me for my help or advice. An example of the latter is when I think of what has been achieved over the past few months. Amongst my recent achievements I count: maintaining my relationships and developing others; learning to live for a year in France and fairly readily slipping back into life in England; improving my French by taking part in French conversations and reading many

French books; generally reading more widely than before in English; learning to cook (although I still have much scope for improvement in this area!) and writing about having Parkinson's.

Another method that I use to help myself if I feel negative is to have aims and to have plans for attaining them. I make my plans detailed so that I can break down what may seem a difficult or complex plan into smaller, simpler sub-plans. Hence, I achieve what I am aiming for, a little at a time, just as I often used to work with people in my career as a psychologist. Examples of my aims for the future are to continue to live half of the year in France and half in England, to make more contacts in England with people who have Parkinson's and, in France, to develop two-way conversation groups for people who want to improve their French or English. I also have plans for further improving my French and becoming an author. I am unlikely to feel negative when I am planning and I have learned repeatedly in life that the best way to guarantee that I don't slide backward is to attempt to move forwards.

It was force of circumstance that brought Jack and I to our current, unusual life-style of living in two countries, but I feel that it has been surprisingly good for my Parkinson's. The most significant benefits can be described under the heading of change. There has been a tendency in me, as the Parkinson's has developed, to hold fast to what I can control and to avoid unpredictability. The danger of this attitude is that it can lead me to become rigid, physically and emotionally. But change is unpredictable and has continually presented me with the antidote to rigidity.

There has been the change of language that forces me to concentrate, particularly carefully, when speaking French; the sense of achievement as my French has improved and the consequent increase in confidence I now feel when speaking in English or French. There are the changes in everyday life routines and expectations. For example, the ordinary courtesies are very different where we live in France: if I go into a French shop in our area it would be very rude of me not to acknowledge everyone present with an appropriate greeting. If I did that in a shop where we live in England I would be viewed as very odd. Similarly, the rituals of shaking hands and embracing have particular rules in France, far more complex than in England.

There are different daily preoccupations to attend to in France than in England. For example, in France there is the septic tank, the wood burning stove in winter, the insects in summer and working out the long lunch time closing sessions of the local shops. In England the importance of awareness of traffic, remembering to lock one's front and back doors, negotiating pavements full of people, and the general high level of background noise become the areas of preoccupation.

Both having Parkinson's and living in two countries have confirmed for me the primary importance of relationships. I am really happy to be making new relationships in France and in England and to have kept my original friends in England. I shall never be able to thank my husband enough for his constant support, his refusal to be perturbed by Parkinson's and for his ingenuity in thinking up new ideas to cope with the surprises that Parkinson's presents. This support, together with my relationships with family and friends, has provided the backbone of my sanity. Luckily, the landline and mobile telephones, texting, e-mailing and visual internet telephone systems mean that one need not feel far away from anyone. That does not provide a substitute for meeting with the people, but it does get near to it.

One often hears that one must learn to accept having Parkinson's and that is no doubt true of any degenerative condition because living in harmony with the disease is far more beneficial than fighting it. However, acceptance cannot be forced and the effort involved in its attainment should not be underestimated. Acceptance comes in its own good time and will mean something different to different people. I think that I prefer the concept of transformation to that of acceptance. By transformation I mean changing what appears to be a negative, difficult situation into a positive, beneficial one. When life presents you with a brick wall, use the bricks to build something new!

16
UNFINISHED BUSINESS

When I completed the previous chapter of this book I thought I had finished writing the book. However now, two years later, I find that I have more to say and so I have started writing again.

Over the past two years my experiences can be contained under two main headings. These are 'Up and Down' and 'Language and Thought'. I shall deal with these topics in the next chapters. However, before doing so I want to give a personal overall impression of the past two years.

First of all, it has been a very happy time. Almost by default I have accepted that I have Parkinson's. I didn't try to do so; it just happened. I can still remember feeling very sad that a part of my life had died, that I could no longer pursue my career or tackle new psychological projects. However, after mourning on and off over a period of about eighteen months, things changed. It was not a question of conscious will power or planning. A significant shift over which I had no control took place in my psyche. If I did manage to influence this shift it was without any conscious understanding of how I did it.

For a long time now I have been using what I call 'creative inactivity' when I am faced with difficult situations that I cannot control. Basically, I try to define my problem, to put it into clear words. Then I make a wish that things will change for the better and I try to believe that this change will happen. I don't have any specific idea of how the problem might be solved; just that alteration in a positive direction can happen and that if it does, I want to be open to recognising it. I call this method, 'creative inactivity' because I don't try to *do* anything about the situation and so one could call the method inactive. The 'creativity' referred to is an openness to all ideas, however incongruous. The fact of wishing may sound strange, but I find it useful in attempting to move from a situation with which I am unhappy, to one where I hope to be happier; not to try to specify how I am going to reach the new situation. The main reason for this is that I have no idea how I will make the change; I only know that it is possible to do so!

What I call 'creative inactivity' is linked with an approach to life which I have found very helpful when I have had a problem to face and when all ideas I have thought of have failed to solve it. The approach basically assumes that doing something about a difficult situation is not necessarily better than doing nothing about it. I had a dream which summarised this for me. In the dream I was in a small boat in a lock. The level of water in which my boat was floating was very low, much lower than the water outside the lock gates. I was feeling depressed in the dream. Then I suddenly realised that if I simply gave the little boat time, it would rise slowly to the level of water outside the lock gates. I did so and stopped feeling depressed.

When I was still mourning the loss of my career I dreamt a lot about the work I used to do and this made me nostalgic, sad and confused about what had happened to me. I dreamt about many of the people with whom I had worked. Now, I can see that I was still saying goodbye to all these people. But the dreams eventually stopped and I began to appreciate the extra time I now had to concentrate on present plans and projects. One of the major improvements to my life was the extra time I was able to spend with people, without having to keep an eye on the clock. Giving up work has meant that I have been able to concentrate more fully on family and friends who have needed my attention and I have felt privileged to be able to do so.

Because I have given up working I have been able to spend more time with my husband, both on our own and in the company of others. Jack has called the time we have spent on our own, 'special' time and I agree with him. There has been a particular quality about it which we would not have known, had we both continued to work.

I have also felt privileged to live in France for six months a year and in England for six months a year. Jack and I propose to continue with this way of life, in which we are regularly exposed to change, as long as we can. Of the different expectations of us to adapt to life in France, the most significant one is that we will speak in French rather than in English. When I go 'down', that is, when my medication is wearing off, my spoken French deteriorates significantly. This disappoints and irritates me but it also emphasises to me the importance of trying to keep developing one's use of language if one has Parkinson's. The deterioration in my language has concerned me a lot and I will enlarge more on this in the next chapter.

Perhaps the discovery which has brought me the most happiness is that my plans and projects have not had to end. They have certainly changed in that they don't involve paid work and I now give myself a lot more time in which to develop them.

However, I have been able to continue to further my aims, which at the time of the previous chapter were: to improve my cooking; to become part of or to develop two-way conversation groups in France; and to meet more people in England who have Parkinson's. Well, the cooking is making progress and we have invited people around frequently for meals. In France, Jack and I help for one afternoon per week in the local library and this has brought us more friends and acquaintances. I cannot overstate the kindness and hospitality which our new French friends have shown us. We have also participated in several small English/ French conversation groups. Then there is the French Parkinson's group which we attend on a monthly basis.

In England we have also joined the local Parkinson's group and have discovered that this is a flourishing organisation which runs many activities and has given us the opportunity to make many new friends. I was initially reluctant to join the group because I was nervous of becoming depressed at meeting other people who might have Parkinson's in a more advanced form than mine. In fact I rapidly became involved, found out how much I was interested in the other people and Jack and I very much appreciate having increased our circle of friends and acquaintances. From September to March, whilst we are in England, there are many activities organised within the Parkinson's group, which we attend. These extend from 'keep fit' in the gym and less formally using the Wii system, to theatre trips and discussion meetings. We also attend a separate Parkinson's singing group called 'Crotchets and Quavers'. This latter group has astounded me inasmuch as I have joined in the fortnightly musical sessions with gusto. I am not exaggerating when I say that mine is not a singing voice one would choose to listen to voluntarily. In the past I have kept it quiet. However, having learned that the muscles which engender speech can be affected by Parkinson's and can be exercised by singing, Jack and I joined this group. My musical ability has not improved, but my confidence at letting my voice rip in public certainly has. I have even sung solo to the group!

I realise that my positive description of the past two years makes it sound as though having Parkinson's doesn't cause me any problems at all and of course that is not true. I have significant difficulties caused by my lack of dopamine and I shall describe them in detail in the next chapter. However, what I have tried to show is that having Parkinson's does not inevitably stop one from being oneself, albeit in a repackaged form, and that one can continue to have a meaningful life by trying new ways of living which, although new, contain the essence of what has always been individual about oneself. I feel that the maintenance of one's sense of self is the most important element in keeping positive despite the progression of Parkinson's Disease.

17
UP AND DOWN

I have had Parkinson's Disease for over ten years now and the main drugs I take at present are Sinemet Plus, Entacapone and Pramipexole.

In Chapter seven I briefly explained what these drugs do to help the person with Parkinson's. However, I shall give another short description here, in order to refresh memories.

Sinemet Plus contains levodopa which is the nearest thing to dopamine that the body has been able to accept so far. Entacapone works with Sinemet Plus to stop the Sinemet Plus from being rapidly broken down by the body. Entacapone cuts down the rate at which levodopa (Sinemet Plus in this case) is destroyed. Pramipexole is a dopamine agonist. This means that it attempts to copy the effects of dopamine even though it is not chemically similar to dopamine in structure.

In Chapter seven I explained the difficult time I experienced in getting used to taking Sinemet Plus. However, after about seven months I started to become accustomed to the drug and things improved a lot for me. First of all, I was no longer experiencing the initial unpleasant side effects of Sinemet Plus and secondly, the drug was starting to do what it was supposed to do: to supplement my low dopamine level so that I was able to return to carrying out many actions that had become very difficult or impossible for me. I was delighted about this, but I soon found out that the positive results of taking levodopa were complicated by the 'on-off' effect. 'On' means that the drug is working and 'off' means that it has stopped working or that it didn't start to work in the first place.

As time has gone on I have found that the 'on-off' effect has become much more intense. My 'ons' are more dramatic than they used to be and my 'offs' are also more extreme, so that I regularly experience two very different states of physical being. At any time I am either 'up' or 'down', 'on' or 'off'. My life is one of predictable change-ability. This sounds like a deliberate contradiction of one term by another. How can changeability be predictable? Well it is, in the fact that when I go 'up' I know I will come 'down' again fairly soon and when I go 'down' I know that I will come 'up' again fairly soon. It is almost like having two bodies: one which is capable and feels quite young; the other which feels old, experiences a lot of discomfort, even pain, moves very slowly and is not physically capable at all.

The following is what happens to me when the dopamine runs out, or perhaps runs low. Professionals call it being 'off'; I refer to it as going 'down':

1. My right arm tightens and becomes painful. So does my right shoulder if I don't rest. My back hurts when I stand. At times the pain is strong.

2. My right arm starts to shake strongly. Then my left arm joins in, although usually not as vigorously.

3. I stoop and move slowly, using laboured steps.

4. At times my head shows a slight involuntary movement.

5. My grip significantly deteriorates so that I cannot write, cut food, manoeuvre food, hold objects such as plates (as in washing up), hold the electric toothbrush to clean my teeth, take coins out of a purse and generally do all the many daily activities which involve holding objects.

6. Any movement tires me, making me more and more clumsy until I simply need to sit down and opt out.

7. My voice becomes quieter and sounds somewhat 'strangled'. Talking tires me and causes me to shake even more.

8. I find it hard to pronounce words and sometimes I produce a lot of saliva, making it harder to say what I want to say.

9. I lose track of what I am saying and this makes me feel foolish so I tend to listen to others rather than speak myself.

10. I can't put the right emphasis into words so that my speech emerges as somewhat of a monotone. I sound uncertain and people tend to help me out with what I am saying.

11. I swerve as I am walking and find it hard to walk in a straight line.

12. I readily lose my balance and feel unsafe unless I hold someone's arm when walking out of doors. This has become more extreme over the past year and I am taking very good care not to fall over.

13. On getting up from a sitting position I am unsteady on my feet and have to concentrate on not falling over.

14. My sight deteriorates in that what I look at appears fuzzy and out of focus.

15. I find it hard to read a book because it shakes in my hands and I can't read the print which is leaping up and down in front of my eyes. I also find it hard to turn the pages because of the shaking.

16. Generally, I find it very difficult to assert myself when I am 'down'.

What about the person who emerges when I switch 'on' or, in my terms, I go 'up'?

The first thing that happens is that I stand up straight. This is a wonderful relief and immediately increases my general feeling of well-being.

Then the following changes occur:

1. The shaking stops.

2. My muscles relax and I no longer have any pain or discomfort.

3. My energy increases.

4. I can write neatly and have even been congratulated for my writing when in this state!

5. I can read a book quite comfortably.

6. I can pick up small objects from flat surfaces.

7. My sight improves.

8. I can take part in a conversation without forgetting my train of thought.

9. I generally feel younger.

In fact, I move from appearing to be a quiet, retiring, stooping and shaking woman to appearing to be a relatively capable, confident, sociable woman. Most people would judge the former person as having some kind of problem, whereas, the latter one would be seen as not particularly out of the ordinary. So, this business of being 'on' or 'off' is accompanied by an apparent personality change. I take my drugs six times per day at present and so I go 'down' six times per day and 'up' six times per day. That is, if the drugs work. So I move from one apparent personality to another personality many times per day. This is not how most people live!

Being a person with Parkinson's involves adjusting to these changes. I don't feel depressed when I go 'down' because I know that I will come up again. Equally, when I am 'up' I have learned not to commit myself to tasks I will probably not be able to fulfil because I know I will go 'down' again. Up and down, up and down are now my daily experiences of life. Somehow, one has to come to terms with this new reality. Somehow, one has to preserve a sense of a continuous self throughout these changes.

What I have found very helpful in trying to integrate these two aspects of 'me' is self knowledge. If I know and understand myself well and can predict how I am likely to feel in the next hour or two, then I won't be in for any nasty surprises and I will feel to some extent in control of myself. This self knowledge depends very much on my understanding of the effects of the drugs I take and of the progression of the illness.

I have a secret weapon for dealing with the situation when I go 'down' in an extreme manner. Sometimes I am not just 'off' or 'down' but 'very off' or 'very down', despite having taken my medication. In this situation the most successful way I have found of maintaining a continuous sense of self is by the sensible use of rest. Rest is my secret weapon. When I am extremely 'down' the only thing which works for me is to rest. I have already explained that Parkinson's does not respect effort or repetition. But it does respond to rest. If I just keep still for thirty minutes or so, abstain from talking and from making any effort at all, then things will improve. But that thirty minutes of doing nothing must be honestly spent in doing nothing. It is no good   continuing a conversation during this time or 'just' tidying a drawer or determinedly dragging myself through some washing up. Nothing means nothing. It means complete rest. Rest implies making a space for oneself, asserting to oneself and to others that one needs to take up this space and then relaxing in it until one comes 'up' again. Whilst resting and relaxing I am not fighting the Parkinson's. I find that this is the only way to deal with the problem of integrating my two states of being, the 'on' and the 'off', the 'up 'and the 'down'. Rest is the most successful activity I have found in managing the most difficult symptoms of Parkinson's. Yes, I realise that that remark is paradoxical!

18
LANGUAGE AND THOUGHT

It has already been mentioned that the condition of Parkinson's can affect one's spoken language. The effect can be extreme in that some people's voices become so quiet that they are difficult or even impossible to understand and eventually they may not be able to vocalise at all. Parkinson's can also affect people's facial muscles, causing these to have limited movement and hence causing their owners' faces to appear nonreactive and blank. This is a particularly difficult effect to deal with because it lessens the ability of the person in question to use non-verbal communication. So, expressions of feelings such as sympathy, joy, excitement, or states of mind such as concentration, interest and distaste are no longer reflected in everyday facial expressions. Instead, the person who has Parkinson's has to live with the indignity of having an impassive, nonreactive face and has to cope with the misjudgement of others, that he or she is at the best uninterested and at the worst, uncaring, heartless and possibly stupid.

For myself, the effect on my language and communication with others is not as apparent or as dramatic as I have described above, but it is significant.

Parkinson's has affected my ability to speak. As with all my symptoms, the strength of the effect depends on where I am in the medication cycle - whether I am 'up' or 'down'.

When I am 'down', I now try to avoid long, detailed or heated conversations. If I do not, my shaking increases, my voice becomes weaker and I become extremely tired. I also find it harder to pronounce words and at times I salivate quite a lot when speaking which makes my words sound unclear.

Language and thought are inextricably interlinked and Parkinson's has affected my thought as well as my language, when I am thinking and talking at the same time. Hence, I am now far less able to hold my own in a discussion, for example. Although it may seem peculiar, I feel that there is a similarity in the way Parkinson's affects my motor movements, my speech and my spoken thought processes. For example, it seems to me that the business of not being able to do more than one thing at a time applies as much to holding thoughts and ideas, as to carrying objects such as books and saucepans.

When I go 'down', my hand grip becomes weak and I can barely hold one object, let alone two. Hence, I drop things. I also become very tired and prefer to sink into an armchair rather than try to continue the physical activity. Similarly, when I go 'down', my ability to pronounce and use words deteriorates. I lose words and, harder to explain, I also lose my direction when I am trying to give an account of an incident or to argue a point. It could be said that my grip on the sentences I am trying to generate becomes tenuous. This feels like my physical tendency to bump into doorways, to lurch and to veer off course when attempting to walk in a straight line. My ability to think out loud is affected in the same way. I tend to launch myself into a conversation and then I lose track of the points I wanted to make; of the direction I was taking. The whole process becomes an enormous effort; I feel my mind going blank and sometimes I feel overwhelmed. Some people finish my sentences for me in these circumstances, but generally I would prefer that they did not. I have recently started to explain to whoever I am with that I can't express myself properly at that time, but that I'll try again later. In fact, I seem to be starting to treat the temporary deterioration in my thinking and language skills as I have been treating my motor skills when they deteriorate. I attempt to use rest until I go 'up' again.

For a long time I have felt that my spatial abilities are affected by Parkinson's. By 'spatial abilities' I mean my ability to keep my body in equilibrium and to maintain a fairly accurate mental map of my surroundings; accurate enough for me to find my way around successfully.

It is self evident that I have lost some of my ability to keep my body in equilibrium because I veer off course when walking; I lurch and lose my balance and I bump into objects. As for maintaining an accurate mental map or representation of my surroundings, this has become more and more difficult. I now find it hard to imagine my surroundings as expressed in map form. My tipping point with regard to this ability happened a few years ago. I was in London and I had to find my way to a particular tube station. I had a street plan but this meant hardly anything to me. I could no longer relate what was on the map to the buildings and streets around me. I decided not to panic and rang Jack on my mobile phone. He talked me to the tube station with the help of an A to Z. I was very relieved, but decided that my days of going into London on my own were over!

Maps are devices to help one get from one place to another; very familiar to most of us is a road map, a drawing which shows the organisation of roads in a particular area. However, unless the map means something to the individual it is of no use. It is clear to me that I have lost much of my ability to read such maps. I wonder whether, when I lose the sequence of what I am saying, the reason may be similar to the above, because my spatial abilities are affected. I think that there is a link between my very poor performance in reading maps, my tendency to veer to one side and to stumble when walking and my loss of a train of thought in conversation. Just as I drop a book because I cannot manage to hold more than one thing at a time, so I 'lose' thoughts, particularly in a long discussion.

So, it seems possible to me that the deterioration in my spatial awareness as regards standing, walking and other movement is linked with the deterioration in my ability to pursue a logical argument.

Thus, Parkinson's continues to surprise me and is far from being simply the shaking disorder that many people perceive it to be.

19
THE FUTURE

I assume that I shall have Parkinson's for the rest of my life. Although much research is being carried out on the condition, I think it unlikely (although I would be very pleased to be proved wrong) that during my lifetime this will have progressed to the extent that people with Parkinson's will receive treatment to regenerate their lost dopamine producing cells. So, I think that Parkinson's is likely to be a constant companion of mine for the remainder of my future. One feature of Parkinson's is that one's condition degenerates with time and so it seems to me that my present, more capable self should take all possible action to help my future self, who will no doubt be far less capable.

When I was very young I thought that it was selfish to put oneself first. I think that I gained this impression as a child, mainly because of the influence of the religion in which I was brought up and later because of the role I ascribed to myself as a woman through society's expectations. But when I became a psychologist and became very involved with counselling, I developed another point of view about 'selfishness'. I realised that a person cannot help other people if they do not first of all look after themselves. We need to take responsibility for knowing ourselves; for understanding our needs and caring for them. We owe this to others as well as to ourselves because squandering our potential is a kind of dishonesty which can lead to depression in ourselves and can infect others. However, learning about ourselves and the course we want to take in life is not always easy or straight forward and often requires the help of close friends, a counsellor, therapist, psychologist or psychiatrist.

In the case of Parkinson's Disease, where individual people's symptoms are often different and where consultants and doctors frequently rely on their patients for information about how they are reacting to a change of medication for example, it is particularly important to know and express one's feelings and needs. Unfortunately, people often shy away from looking at themselves honestly because they are reluctant to accept some aspects of their personalities. Yet, none of us can help what we feel and far more harm can be done by hiding from what we may consider to be unacceptable, than by facing it.

Recently, I have been trying to take a good look at some of the ways my Parkinson's might develop in the future and how I can help that future self from my vantage point now. One of my current concerns about the future is to prepare for the time when my drugs become less effective. I am extremely grateful for the anti-Parkinson's drugs which I have taken in increasing quantities over the past few years; they have undoubtedly improved my quality of life immeasurably and I realise that life would have been very difficult without them. *How* difficult is graphically described by James Parkinson in *'An essay on the Shaking Palsy'* written in 1817 and easily obtainable on the Internet. The people described by James Parkinson were in a pitiful state.

In time, people usually develop a tolerance to anti-Parkinson's drugs. This means that after a while the drugs cease to work effectively and one has to take higher and higher dosages to achieve the same result. Unfortunately, taking greater quantities of anti-Parkinson's drugs makes it more likely that severe side effects such as dyskinesias and hallucinations will show themselves. So far, I have not experienced hallucinations as a result of taking my medication. However, I have recently become aware of dyskinesias. Dyskinesias are involuntary movements of parts of the body, including the limbs and the head, which often arise in a person with Parkinson's several years after they have started to take levodopa (in my case, Sinemet Plus). My experiences of dyskinesias have started with movements of my right foot. I get a kind of hyperactive feeling in this foot at times and then it spreads to other areas of my body, causing the different parts to move. When I am talking enthusiastically, my foot, leg, arms and head bob around and my body sways a little from side to side. I can control these movements when I concentrate on them, but when I am not thinking about them they increase.

However, I have met people with far more severe dyskinesias than mine, who cannot control these movements at all. The constant movement of one's limbs can become tiring, embarrassing and depressing. The dyskinesias can hinder everyday actions such as eating and can stop the person concerned from focussing on anything which demands stillness or control of fine motor movements.

Another symptom which has just started for me is that of occasional memory loss. The French call it, 'trous de mémoire' (holes in the memory). I have recently experienced a few occasions when I have totally forgotten something which has happened a short time ago, although I have eventually remembered when I have been reminded. This loss of memory and the onset of dyskinesias have coincided with an increase in my dosage of drugs.

These experiences suggest to me that there is a price to pay for the dramatic improvements in my movements brought about by the medication I have been taking over the years. These improvements allow me to move far more freely than I did a few years ago. I remember four years ago, following Jack around IKEA in France: I felt exhausted; I had pains in my arm; I was shaking, stooping and generally felt very ill. I was embarrassed at visiting the toilet because I shook so much whilst waiting in the inevitable queue. In contrast, I can now visit shops, including their toilets and generally feel comfortable, so long as I have taken my medication, of course. Also, if I am very careful with the timing of my medication, I can usually avoid having a major shaking attack in a particular social or formal situation. However, now I sway and lose parts of my memory! This is probably the price worth paying.

I have described the dramatic effects of the drugs I

currently take. However, I am very dependent on them and it is important not to forget that the cruel side of Parkinson's is only just around the corner; just a few pills away. This cruel side shows itself when I take the tablets late or when they don't work. When I am 'very down' I feel ill. My walking, talking, muscular ability, sight and balance all deteriorate very rapidly. I become exhausted and cannot easily maintain a train of thought in conversation. I can also develop strong pains at these times which seem to be indiscriminate in their choice of where to attack. I have had these pains in my shoulders, legs and back and although they can be kept under control by constant rubbing, moving and stretching, they only really improve when I can take more of that wonderful drug, Sinemet Plus.

I am aware that a lot of research is under way to find new anti-Parkinson's drugs and I think that in the near future there are likely to be startling developments in this area of treatment. Two of the most recent drugs which I have been taking have made a lot of difference for me as my Parkinson's has developed. They are Entacapone and Pramipexole. Entacapone slows the breakdown of levodopa, which I take in the form of Sinemet Plus. The effect I notice is that my 'up' times are about 30 minutes longer when I take Entacapone at the same time as Sinemet Plus. The Pramipexole gives me an overall feeling of greater energy and well being. Taking my cocktail of Levodopa, Entacapone and Pramipexole helps me to feel generally far better today than I felt three or four years ago. This does depend on being very careful about timing the medication accurately, which again relies on monitoring my response to the drugs.

Looking to my future, it is likely that my symptoms will increase, but that after a time I will not be able to continue increasing the amount of levodopa that I will need because of the interference of the side effects mentioned above. By that time it will be important that I have taken every opportunity to try alternative drugs or treatments which could help the situation. During my last two visits to my Consultant, whom I see every six months, she has suggested that I consider having a brain operation which could help my symptoms and which would probably result in my taking less anti-Parkinson's drugs, hence less chance of the dyskinesias, hallucinations and other problems.

The brain operation concerned is called Deep Brain Stimulation or DBS. According to the literature this is a largely successful operation which can lessen the tremors and rigidity of Parkinson's and can result in the patient needing less anti-Parkinson's drugs. However, there are risks; the operation involves having one or more electrodes implanted into one's brain, wires under the skin which run from the electrodes to the chest and a small battery implanted in the chest. One danger is that the electrodes might cause a stroke, which in itself could cause paralysis and speech problems. Another concern of mine is the possibility of infection which is present when any operation is carried out, let alone on the brain. So, I am currently thinking hard about the pros and cons of DBS.

Another suggestion, which has been put to me by my consultant, is the self injection of apomorphine. Apomorphine is a dopamine agonist which is injected directly into the blood stream. Apparently, it is the strongest of the dopamine agonists so far and acts fast when it is injected, but only for a short time, around forty minutes to an hour. As far as I understand, self injection of apomorphine is a convenient way of alleviating one's symptoms on a temporary basis when they become overpowering. The problem about being injected regularly is the danger of developing infection around the sites of the injections. There is another way of administering apomorphine which is by having a small pump attached to one's body and for the pump to administer regular doses of the drug. This can also cause infection.

However, looking after oneself does not only involve drugs and operations.

Alternative approaches such as relaxation, meditation, hypnosis and shiatsu can help one's overall sense of well being and can encourage or maintain one's positivity. I have only recently encountered shiatsu and I am hopeful about its benefit. Shiatsu involves pulling and stretching the arms and legs as well as applying pressure to various key parts of the body. I have a friend in France who is a shiatsu practitioner and she is about to include me in a survey on the effects of shiatsu on Parkinson's .

I believe that looking after oneself, above all, involves

developing one's sense of self. I use this term to describe a person who has developed a clear perception of who they are, who accepts themselves, who values themselves and who attempts to fulfil their potential as far as possible. I am quite aware that this is a very difficult state to achieve. The advantage of being older is that we know ourselves, our abilities and our weak points better than when we were younger. The disadvantage is that we are more limited, both physically and intellectually. And of course, Parkinson's adds to those limitations, in variety as well as intensity.

Looking after oneself also involves having successful relationships with other people. If I had to choose between not having relationships and not having Parkinson's I would opt for keeping the Parkinson's. We are used to saying that we come into this world on our own and that we leave it on our own. That sounds a likely assumption, but for whatever time we spend in this world we are not on our own. We have other people to relate to. The most important thing in this life, as far as I am concerned, is trying to understand other people. That is why I became a psychologist. When I was very young I was convinced that mental suffering is worse than physical suffering and, with some exceptions, I still think so. My view of some mental suffering, put very simply, is that it occurs when a person loses the sense of who they are and when the way the person lives their life is at odds with the way that they would follow, if they were being true to themselves. Losing the sense of self can be catastrophic, causing depression, chronic anxiety and episodes of serious emotional disturbance. It should be added, however, that the outcomes of such 'breakdowns' can be very positive if the appropriate help is provided.

My purposes in life are particular to me. The point is that they have not changed because I have Parkinson's. I am definitely not suggesting that other people try to copy my view of life or my aims. What I am trying to say is that everyone has a responsibility to attempt to develop themselves, even if they have Parkinson's, and that people's purposes in life do not have to change because they develop Parkinson's.

When I started writing this book I said that when I first knew I had Parkinson's I did not know what to feel because I did not know what to expect. Well now, after over ten years of Parkinson's, I have some idea of what to expect and I have tried to describe my experiences in some detail in case they are helpful for others. As regards my feelings, they are tied up with the degree of fulfilment I experience as a human being. In fact, Parkinson's has helped me because it has emphasised that having this condition is less important to me than who I am, what I am doing and how I relate with others. Having Parkinson's can be very difficult at times and sometimes it can cause me to lose my way for a while, but when all is said and done it has not altered my perception of who I am and what I am aiming for and that is good enough for me.

ADDENDUM
PRACTICAL APPROACHES

Together with the examples that I have given in Chapter four, these are methods that I have evolved for meeting practical difficulties. If I have already addressed them in Chapter four I have indicated so. These methods work for me, but they may not all help other people:

PUTTING ON A JACKET, CARDIGAN ETC...
Ways of tackling it:
Put 'worse' arm in first, struggle for a little while and then ask for help, if necessary. If there is no one to ask, lay the garment on its back on a bed (so that the inside lining can be seen) and stretch the sleeves out. Then sit on the bed, put one arm at a time into the garment and pull it on.

PUTTING ON GLOVES, INCLUDING RUBBER GLOVES.
Ways of tackling it:
Surprisingly, I have found that for gloves, I have to put the 'best' hand in first.

DRESSING.
Ways of tackling it:
See Chapter four. It takes me a long time to wash or shower and dress in the mornings; about an hour. Zips and buttons are difficult and Velcro can be very useful. I feel that it is important to take my time when getting dressed and not be rushed, to give me a calm start to the day. I

continue to find a full-length mirror of great use.

UNDRESSING.
Ways of tackling it:
See Chapter four.

USING A FACE FLANNEL.
Ways of tackling it:
Use a glove flannel; have baths or showers rather than overall washes; have a bidet installed.

TEETH CLEANING.
Ways of tackling it:
This has become impossible for me unless I use an electric toothbrush. The repetitive movements involved in non-electric teeth cleaning bring my movement to a speedy halt.

SALIVA AND PLAQUE.
Ways of tackling it:
This sounds a horrible topic but must be faced! The drugs I take cause my saliva to go brown during my sleep. When I wake up my pillowslip is stained and so I change it every day. In addition, they cause my mouth to become extremely dry, particularly during sleep. This causes a build up of plaque in my mouth and at one time I was embarrassed to go to the dentist because it must have seemed that I never cleaned my teeth, although I was doing so at least four times per day. However, I have found it very useful to rinse my mouth out several times with hot

water if I wake up in the night or early morning. This has improved the plaque problem.

WASHING MY HAIR.
Ways of tackling it:
I can't wash my hair in the bowl but I can do it in the shower. I may soon need a stool to sit on in the shower.

BLOW DRYING MY HAIR.
Ways of tackling it:
Jack kindly does this. Occasionally, I go to the hairdresser and I do find it stressful to have to sit still for the amount of time necessary. I ensure that the hairdresser knows that I have Parkinson's and I try to relax to minimise the shaking.

PUTTING ON FACE CREAM.
Ways of tackling it:
If I use my hands separately the right one tends to stop moving. However, if I use them together the right hand joins in with the left, rather like when I am typing.

GETTING INTO AND OUT OF BED.
Ways of tackling it:
I have found that either a very high or a very low bed suits me best. A very high one means that I can get into or out of bed in an almost sitting position. A very low one means that I can use my all-fours manoeuvre.

CUTTING FINGER AND TOE NAILS.
Ways of tackling it:
Unfortunately, I can't do this for myself but I can file my nails, although the effect of repetitive movement can make my filing ineffective.

GETTING OUT OF THE BATH.
Ways of tackling it:
I use the all-fours technique. However, recently I have had a lot less difficulty with getting out of the bath, since my medication has been increased.

WASHING SMALL GARMENTS BY HAND.
Ways of tackling it:
During my pre-Parkinson's life I sometimes found it useful to be able to wash small pieces of underwear by hand. However, the repetitive movements involved in washing clothes now make this very difficult for me. Instead, whilst waiting for a machine load, I ensure that I always have several 'spares' available. So, I buy far more underwear than before!

PULLING UP PANTS AND TROUSERS.
Ways of tackling it:
I find this particularly difficult when using public toilets, for the reasons given earlier. I try to keep relaxed, encourage myself (mentally, if I can be over heard!) and count 'one, two, three' with the actions I am trying to carry out. This 'self-talk' really helps.

PUTTING ON TIGHTS.
Ways of tackling it:
Impossible! The only time I will consent to wear tights again is if the Royal Family ask me round for tea. In that case I shall hire a couple of helpers and ask them to fit my tights onto me. The fine motor skills involved in putting on a pair of tights must be at least equivalent to playing the violin! The last time I tried (unsuccessfully) to put on a pair of tights I had to rest for more than half an hour to get over the ordeal.

GETTING OUT OF A CHAIR.
Ways of tackling it:
I try to sit in as high a chair as possible. If the chair is low, I manoeuvre myself to the edge of the chair and try to get up; if this doesn't work I ask someone for a slight push (not a pull); if that doesn't work I sink onto all fours and get up that way. However, since my levodopa has been increased I have far less difficulty in getting up from a sitting position.

GETTING OUT OF A CAR.
Ways of tackling it:
I try always to get out of the left side of the car because my right side is my 'worse' side and the least helpful in lifting me.

PUTTING ON A SAFETY BELT IN A CAR.
Ways of tackling it:
Similarly, I sit on the left side of the car and use my left

hand to manoeuvre the safety belt. I sometimes need help.

SHOPPING FOR CLOTHES.
Ways of tackling it:
It has become too exhausting to go shopping for clothes; merely trying on one garment finishes me off. Instead, I use catalogues or else I buy from shops that have an easy returns policy and then I try on the garments at home. Incidentally, I feel that it is extremely important for my self-esteem that I continue to try to look as presentable as possible and I continue to enjoy buying new clothes.

SHOPPING FOR FOOD AND SIMILAR ITEMS.
Ways of tackling it:
I can do this, but only after detailed planning as follows:

1) Have a clear list with items grouped according to where they are to be bought. If visiting a supermarket I try to get to know where the items will be in the shop and group them accordingly.

2) If a trolley is available in the shop I use one even if I am buying a small number of items. Trolleys can prop me up if I am not walking steadily or become tired. They are also useful when trying to hide shaking in that one can move one's hands around much more easily to do so.

3) If I have to carry shopping home I am very conservative in my estimate of how much I can carry.

4) If offered help in packing shopping I always take it. If not offered help I tell the check out person that I have Parkinson's, to explain my snail like speed. With luck, I

am then offered help.

5) My preferred method of paying is with a plastic card that has a PIN number. Signing is now out of the question, apart from at a good time that cannot be predicted. If I have to pay by cash, I ensure that I know exactly what is in my purse. However, I may have to ask for help in retrieving coins and notes from the purse.

READING.
Ways of tackling it:
When the medication isn't working and I am shaking I sit at a table to read so that I can hold the pages down with other books or objects such as table mats. Also, the print needs to be clear and the lighting has to be bright in order to compensate for the constant up and down motion.

Recently, I was given an electronic book, a Kindle, and this has transformed my life. I can adjust the size of the print on the Kindle; it will store about three thousand books; it is light to carry and turning pages involves a mere press of a button. It is far easier to read than an ordinary book.

WRITING.
Ways of tackling it:
As I have already described, the only time I can write legibly is around an hour and a quarter after taking levodopa. This window of writing legibility lasts for about twenty minutes and so I keep birthday cards, things which need signing, short notes to write etc... for these occasions.

TYPING AND GENERALLY USING A COMPUTER.
Ways of tackling it:
Thank heavens for computers. However, I have to guard against using my 'good' hand all the time. The danger is that the worse hand can become increasingly useless because it is not used. Also the dexterity of the worse hand improves when it is used together with the good hand.

TELEPHONE (LAND LINE).
Ways of tackling it:
When I hold the phone to my ear it bounces up and down against my ear. This impedes my hearing and my arm becomes tired, stiff and painful when the call goes on for a few minutes. The simplest solution has been to wear headphones which have freed both my hands. Another answer has been to use 'Skype', an internet telephone system where one uses the computer, microphone and speaker. This is excellent and it is downloadable, free, from the internet. If the computer incorporates a camera, one can also communicate using visual means. However, to use Skype free of charge, the person I am speaking to also has to have Skype.

MOBILE PHONE.
Ways of tackling it:
Because my hands shake so much I invariably press the keys more than once or I press the wrong keys. It then takes a long time to erase my mistakes, and to rewrite, especially when texting. I find that 'dragging' pages on my mobile phone is easier than pressing buttons. I am going to

find out about voice activated mobile phones. See page 65, Chapter eleven.

EATING.
Ways of tackling it:
I mentioned various ways of tackling this in Chapter four. The eating problem has worsened for me and if I am going out for a meal, whether to a restaurant or to someone's home, I pay great attention to the timing of my medication, trying to achieve an 'on' period for the meal. I try not to tackle any food which needs cutting, including salad, and as I have mentioned previously, I use my fingers to eat with at times and I am still absolutely delighted if I am served up risotto.

DRINKING.
Ways of tackling it:
My shaking results in a clacking sound as the cup or glass rattles against my spectacles. The answer is to take my spectacles off or to drink from a receptacle with a wider rim. I have also found that I have to tip my head back further than I used to, in order to swallow. Using a straw can be very useful when the shaking becomes extremely enthusiastic.

WALKING.
Ways of tackling it:
As the Parkinson's progresses I find that I am becoming less balanced when I walk, especially when I turn and also

when I stand up from a sitting position. When I am out of doors I always walk with someone and preferably take the person's arm, in case of veering or stumbling. Several people with Parkinson's whom I know have fallen without warning and I want to avoid that, if I can.

When moving from one environment (for example, a room) to another (for example, a corridor) I try to hold onto something or someone to steady myself because such a transition can cause me to swerve quite dangerously.

I never stand too near to the edge of the platform in the underground. The relative speed of the train compared with my stationary position makes me dangerously unsteady. Even worse, however, is when I am walking along the platform and the train arrives. To keep safe I stand back from the train until it has stopped and the doors have opened.

PUBLIC TRANSPORT.
Ways of tackling it:
I have found that people are very kind to me on public transport. I am invariably offered a seat in packed buses and train carriages. Men, women and children of all sizes, ages and ethnicity get up and offer me their seats. I always accept the offer, thank the person concerned and sit down gratefully.

CARRYING.
Ways of tackling it:
My problem is not in the weight of what I carry, but in my dexterity. If I carry more than one thing at a time I am

likely to drop one and so I keep to the one item rule, even if this means that I have to make more journeys.

DROPPING THINGS.
Ways of tackling it:
As my Parkinson's progresses I am becoming clumsier and I frequently drop things. This is inconvenient and occasionally dangerous. My strategy for overcoming this is caution. I have to be very careful and I have to resist any verbal or non-verbal encouragements to 'hurry up'. I can't hurry up. I've got Parkinson's!

HURRYING MY SPEECH.
Ways of tackling it:
I have explained that my language has deteriorated, both in pronouncing words and in following a train of thought. I have to be given time to achieve what I am trying to say. People who finish my sentences for me usually mean to be kind, but they may misunderstand what I intended to say and I feel quite inadequate.

PLANNING.
Ways of tackling it:
All the above practical strategies depend on planning how to cater for the situation. With Parkinson's, planning makes things much better and not planning can cause things to go very wrong.

PERSEVERING WITH PHYSICAL TASKS.
Ways of tackling it:
Talking to myself 'in my head' or out loud if I am on my own, helps me to persevere with physical tasks that I find difficult, especially dressing. I count 'one, two, three' or say 'well done, you're getting there' and other such encouraging phrases.

REMEMBERING TO TAKE MY DRUGS ON TIME.
Ways of tackling it:
Timing of drugs is very important for people with Parkinson's. It an cause the difference between 'staying up' and becoming 'very down'.
Most recently I have six sessions of drug-taking per day and I would forget the times and details of these, were it not for my memo book. This is a little notebook with attached pencil which I keep in my handbag. At the beginning of each day I count out my tablets for that day and use the notebook to write what I am to take, at what time and record when I have done so.
I use a pill box. There are a lot of these on the market and they make good presents for people who have to take a lot of medication.